Addiction-Free
Naturally

Addiction-Free
Naturally

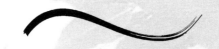

Liberating Yourself from

SUGAR • CAFFEINE
FOOD ADDICTIONS
TOBACCO • ALCOHOL
PRESCRIPTION DRUGS

BRIGITTE MARS
HERBALIST AHG

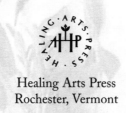

Healing Arts Press
Rochester, Vermont

To Ronnie, Steve, Kay, Sergai, and Shannon

Healing Arts Press
One Park Street
Rochester, Vermont 05767
www.InnerTraditions.com

Healing Arts Press is a division of Inner Traditions International

Note to the reader: This book is intended as an informational guide. The remedies, approaches, and techniques described herein are meant to supplement, and not to be a substitute for, professional medical care or treatment. They should not be used to treat a serious ailment without prior consultation with a qualified health care professional.

Library of Congress Cataloging-in-Publication Data

Mars, Brigitte.
    Addiction-free naturally : liberating yourself from sugar, caffeine, food
addictions, tobacco, alcohol, and prescription drugs / Brigitte Mars.
      p. cm.
    Includes bibliographical references and index.
    ISBN 0-89281-892-1 (alk. paper)
      1. Substance abuse—Alternative treatment. 2. Compulsive behavior—
Patients—Rehabilitation. 3. Compulsive behavior—Treatment. 4. Addicts—
Rehabilitation. I. Title.

RC564 .M298 2001
616.86'06—dc21
                                                                    00-039577

Printed and bound in Canada

10 9 8 7 6 5 4 3 2 1

Text design and layout by Virginia Scott-Bowman
This book was typeset in Caslon with Aldus and Felix Titling as the display typefaces

Contents

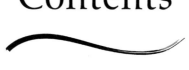

Acknowledgments

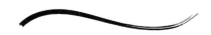

Thank you to my editor, Lee Juvan, for seeing the need for this book, and to Nancy Ringer for her eagle-eyed attention to the text. Thanks to my beloved Tom Pfeiffer, who had to put up with me being a workaholic while writing and brought me lovely yerba matés to keep me going. Thank you to Matthew Becker for great talks and always having a sound answer to my many questions; and to Mindy Green, my dear friend, who lets me tap into her great stores of knowledge.

PART ONE

Natural and Herbal
Approaches to Treating Addiction

1

Facing the Facts
Coming to Terms
with Addiction

No other disease affects as many people as addiction. Current estimates suggest that addictions affect one-third of the population in
the United States; that's one in three people who are addicted or are
directly involved with an addict. Of course, when most of us hear the
word *addict*, we think crack, or cocaine, or heroin, or any of the other
horrifyingly addictive illegal street drugs we've been teaching our
children to abhor. Certainly we don't think about, say, sugar—and yet
sugar is the most prevalent addictive substance in the world!

As a society we're well schooled on what constitutes an addiction, as
well as what does not. The United States' "war on drugs" is not about
getting office workers to ease back on coffee, though perhaps it should
be—caffeine has been linked to anxiety, depression, insomnia, fibrocystic breast disease, cardiovascular disease, birth defects, and reproductive problems, and, as you've probably found out for yourself, it's
highly addictive. When our schoolchildren wear T-shirts emblazoned
JUST SAY NO, they're not talking about chocolate—although it can
stunt their growth and cause fatigue, hyperactivity, obesity, depression,

acne, heartburn, and heart disease. And, yes, chocolate works just like an addictive drug—it stimulates feel-good neurotransmitters, and when these effects wear off, it leaves us wanting more.

Addiction-Free—Naturally addresses what could be called societal addictions: the addictive substances that have wormed their way into the daily life of Western culture. I'm not talking about smoking dope here; I'm talking about that habitual morning cup of coffee, about cigarette breaks, about refined sugar being a major ingredient in just about every packaged food on the market. Addictions are endemic to our society. Some of us are fortunate enough to avoid them. Some of us know we have addictions, and we try time and time again to kick them. Others of us have simply yet to see the warning signs.

No substance is all good or all bad. As the old proverb says, "The evil lies within the man, not the drug." Most addictive substances have significant and valuable applications. We know these uses, and we know the dangers inherent to them. If we ignore the dangers, we must take responsibility for our decisions. Addiction is our own self-made malaise. We have created it, and we are the only ones who can overcome it.

Having an addiction does not make you a bad or weak-willed person. Indeed, addictions are quite common; more people have them than not. Some addictions are a self-destructive response to life stressors. Others are a natural by-product of the society we live in. The important thing—and often the most difficult thing—is to realize and acknowledge an addiction. Once you've taken that first step, you're well on your way to beating it.

The Quest for Purity

Throughout history virtually every culture has devised some way of altering consciousness, whether it be through fermented fruit or grain, mushrooms, or tobacco. Alcohol, tobacco, and various other mind-bending substances were traditionally used for medicine, ceremony, and celebration. In past ages addiction was considered a mortal sin and was treated with ridicule, punishment, and even exorcism.

Are You Addicted?

1. Do you feel that you just don't want to stop indulging in a particular substance—caffeine, sugar, tobacco, alcohol—right now, although you could at any time?
2. Have you ever tried to stop for a week but been unable to do so?
3. Do you resent the advice of others who express concern about your substance use?
4. Have you ever tried to control your addiction by switching to an alternative addictive substance? For instance, have you ever taken up smoking so that you could give up drinking?
5. Do you envy people who can indulge without getting into trouble?
6. Has your substance use created problems with friends and family?
7. Do you try to avoid family or friends when you're using your substance?
8. Have you lost relationships because of substance abuse?
9. Are your friendships determined by whether others indulge in the same substances as you?
10. Do you indulge in your substance alone?
11. Have you ever neglected your family or work for more than two days in a row due to substance abuse?
12. When substances are limited or unavailable at social events, do you try to obtain some anyway?
13. Have you missed time from work during the past year due to substance use?
14. Has your substance of choice stopped being fun to use?
15. When you are low on your substance, do you feel anxious or worried about how to get more?
16. Do you plan your life around your substance use?
17. Do you ever consume more of your particular substance than you intend to?
18. Are you consuming more than you used to in order to feel the same effects?
19. Do you consume as much as you can and feel reluctant to discard any leftovers?
20. Are you experiencing financial difficulty due to substance use?

21. Do you use your substance when you are disappointed, depressed, or going through a difficult time?

22 Does your substance use affect your sleep?

23. Has your sexual ability or desire suffered from your substance use?

24. Are you concerned that if you stop using, you will lack energy, motivation, confidence, or the ability to relax?

25. Do you use your substance repeatedly to sleep or stay awake?

26. Do you ever lie to others about how much or how often you consume your particular substance?

27. Have you ever stolen money or goods to support your habit?

28. Have you lost a job because of substance use?

29. Do you ever regret the way you behaved while you were on a substance-use high?

30. Do you experience irritability, headaches, or tremors when you have not consumed your particular substance for a while?

31. Have you ever passed out from substance use?

32. Have you ever felt your life would be more productive if you were not indulging in that particular substance?

33. Have you become more irritable and difficult to get along with?

34. Is your pattern of use potentially dangerous? (This can be true even in cases where substance consumption is neither frequent nor excessive.)

35. Do you lack self-control in deciding whether or not to consume your particular substance?

36. Is your habit putting you into a state of poor health?

37. Is your substance abuse dangerous to others? (Via secondhand smoke, drunk driving, using up family resources, et cetera?)

How many questions did you answer *yes* to? Deep down inside, if you are being honest with yourself, you know if you have a substance-abuse problem or are on your way to one. Do something about it now, while you can.

When the world of medicine changed, however, it changed fast. In the nineteenth century active plant ingredients were discovered and isolated in quick succession—morphine in 1806, codeine in 1832, atropine in 1833, caffeine in 1841, cocaine in 1860, heroin in 1883, and mescaline in 1896.

Addictive substances began to become a greater part of society. By 1850, for example, sugar (99.5 percent sucrose) became widely available and very cheap. And in the 1860s alcohol and narcotics replaced calomel (made from mercury) and bleeding as the vogue medical treatments. Though that may not sound like a big improvement, it was: at least alcohol and narcotics killed you slowly, rather than quickly, and if you managed to stop taking them before the end, they actually could do you some good.

Chemists became obsessed with extracting active ingredients from plants. Somehow it just seemed more scientific and modern to turn everything into a white powder: cocaine, heroin, and for that matter white sugar and flour. Medicine embarked on a quest for purity. Dried green plants seemed too plain and primitive—and less profitable.

The more refined a substance becomes, the more likely it is to have side effects and addictive tendencies. Plants are a symphony of structure and wonder—vitamins, minerals, essential oils, blood-building chlorophyll, saponins, glycosides, alkaloids, and more. They are not meant to be refined. Take, for example, opium. It has traditional use in folk medicine as a sedative and soporific, and it's only mildly addictive; once refined to a white crystalline form, however, it becomes heroin, a highly addictive substance with incredibly dangerous side effects.

It was not until after World War II that addiction was recognized as a legitimate disease.

Why Addiction Occurs

Why do some people find themselves frequently indulging in things that they know are not good for them, while others are able to exercise restraint without struggling? Many addictions have their roots in painful childhood experiences. According to a study undertaken by the National Academy of Sciences, children are more likely to end up addicted to something if they are physically abused, humiliated, or lied to, and if their parents are themselves substance abusers. For example, alcoholism is four to five times more prevalent among the biological children of alcoholics than among those with nonalcoholic parents.

New research suggests that we may well be hardwired for addiction from a very tender age. Specific signs point to children at risk. Bottle-fed children with learning disabilities or attention deficit disorder who eat excessive amounts of sugary foods and receive little guidance in accepting responsibility are at higher risk of developing allergies, diabetes, and addictive tendencies. Deprivation or overindulgence and shifts between excessive praise and discipline during childhood can also contribute to addiction in adulthood.

Children in the United States often begin experimenting with drugs and alcohol as early as the fourth grade. In the lower grades they are more likely to try substances to feel older, in the middle grades to fit in, and in the upper grades for a good time. Young people who have little interest in spiritual values or academic goals and lack parental support are at the highest risk for drug abuse. Those who share a close relationship with family members and feel a part of a loving community are less likely to get into trouble with substance abuse. Families can help keep their children from developing danger-ous addictions by establishing good communication patterns early on and helping their children set realistic goals for the future. The old saying is true: "Teach your children well!"

Still, even those with relatively uneventful childhoods can grow into adults with emotional imbalances. Who doesn't have a mustard seed of insecurity hidden away inside? As children we were afraid of the monsters under the bed, and as adults we give the monsters new names: financial insecurity, relationship problems, job stress. All stem from fear of the unknown and fear of change. If loneliness, rejection, self-destruction, hostility, anxiety, and stress are the seeds firmly planted in our psyches, then fear is the water and sunshine that helps addiction spring up. Not feeling adequately loved and not being able to express our true feelings, dreams, and fears can set us up for hard times and open the door to substance abuse.

Biological Factors in Addiction

Many biological factors can contribute to addictions, including low thyroid function, poor adrenal function, malfunctioning neurotransmitters, nutritional deficiencies, adrenal insufficiency, fatigue, and yeast overgrowth. Two of the most common are hypoglycemia and food allergies.

The correlation between hypoglycemia and addiction is indisputable. The question is which causes which. It's known that hypoglycemics have a strong reaction to simple sugars, such as those found in food and alcohol. And many addictive substances, including tobacco, alcohol, and sugar, raise blood sugar levels, which over time can lead to hypoglycemia. So does hypoglycemia make you more prone to developing addictions, or is it the addiction that makes you hypoglycemic? It's likely to be a little of both. What's interesting is that symptoms of hypoglycemia are the same as symptoms of addiction: irritability, restlessness, fatigue, anxiety, depression, confusion, sluggish thinking, emotional outbursts, and negativity.

Hypoglycemia can play a part in antisocial behavior as well. According to Michio Kushi, author of *Crime and Diet: The Macrobiotic Approach*, as much as 80 to 85 percent of our prison population is hypoglycemic.

Allergies can also be major factors in addictive behavior. If you consume a food to which you are allergic or sensitive, you may initially experience an increase in metabolism, causing an energy rush. As this feeling wears off and you return to normal, you feel a decrease in energy, which leads to a craving for the food that stimulated that high. Allergies are frequently the culprit behind food addictions and can even stimulate alcohol addictions, because the grains used to make alcohol—wheat, rye, and barley—are common allergens.

The Chemistry of Addiction

The human brain is composed of about one hundred billion neurons. Neurons are nerve cells that consist of a body, an axon (or spine), and dendrites, which extend like branches from a tree from the neuron body. Although billions of neurons are packed into the brain, they never touch. The small gaps between them are called synapses. To send signals across neurons, the brain uses neurotransmitters, chemical messengers that cross the synapses and attach

In 1853 the hypodermic syringe was invented by the Scottish physician Alexander Wood. His wife became the first morphine addict.

themselves to receptor sites embedded in the dendrites.

The relationship between receptors and neurotransmitters is often compared to that of a lock and key. The receptor site is like a lock that can be opened only with the proper chemical key. Only neurotransmitters with the proper shape will fit into that lock. However, substances with shapes similar to that of the familiar neurotransmitter can trick the receptor and dock at that site, thereby blocking access for the neurotransmitter. Some addictive substances work in this fashion, crossing the blood-brain barrier into the brain and mimicking the effects of neurotransmitters. Other addictive substances stimulate or inhibit the production and transmission of neurotransmitters to influence mood.

⁓

The body's autonomic nervous system is divided into two parts: the sympathetic and the parasympathetic nervous systems. The sympathetic nervous system (SNS) contains chiefly adrenergic (activated by epinephrine, also called adrenaline) fibers and increases heart rate. When a fight-or-flight reaction kicks in—heart racing, rapid breathing, acute sensory input—it's the sympathetic nervous system that's in charge. The SNS is our workhorse, what motivates us to explore, discover, and master. The SNS employs the neurotransmitters norepinephrine and epinephrine.

The parasympathetic nervous system (PSNS) contains chiefly cholinergic (activated by acetylcholine) fibers and slows heart rate. It's often referred to as the "feed-and-breed" system, because it governs our drive for natural functions such as eating, drinking, sleeping, elimination, and reproduction. The PSNS is what motivates us to rest, recuperate, and rebuild.

Each part of the nervous system has its own pleasure incentive, ensuring that we can work and recover. Activation of the SNS induces release of dopamine, which lifts the spirits and makes us feel energized. Activation of the PSNS induces release of endorphins, which have an analgesic effect and help us feel calm and satisfied. The sympathetic-parasympathetic dance of energy governs our behavior. For example, when endorphins are elevated, we are motivated to eat (which in itself triggers further endorphin release); when dopamine levels are elevated, we are motivated not to eat.

The feelings of well-being that neurotransmitters can induce are a large part of what attracts us to addictive substances. For example, alcohol, sugar, and many types of drugs stimulate the parasympathetic nervous system. Other drugs, such as amphetamines, stimulate the sympathetic nervous system. The resulting chemical imbalance disrupts all of our natural functions and affects our mood, energy, temperament, sleep, and health. The body tries to compensate. When we give it stimulants, it cuts back on dopamine production. When we use sedatives, endorphin production is diminished. As we become more and more out of balance, we begin to depend on outside stimulants to induce what used to be natural reactions. When we begin to crave those outside stimulants, the addiction cycle has closed around us.

Get to Know Your Neurotransmitters

The neurotransmitters most involved with addictions are dopamine, endorphins, enkephalin, epinephrine (adrenaline) and norepinephrine, GABA (gamma-aminobutyric acid), and serotonin.

Eastern Perspectives on Addiction

According to the principles of traditional Chinese medicine (TCM), addictions cause stagnation of chi (life force) in the liver. The liver cleanses the body of negative emotions, and chi stagnation in the liver contributes to feelings of anger and stunts creativity.

Addictions also cause kidney and adrenal stress, which leads to coldness in the body, frequent urination, and jing (vital essence) deficiency. TCM holds that when the kidneys are weak, the brain also becomes weak.

Addiction causes derangement in the heart-mind-spirit connection, contributing to lack of concentration, agitation, and sleep disorders as well as general deficiency causing lack of motivation, energy, paleness, thinness, and lack of appetite. Addiction also causes a deficiency in chi because the abuser focuses on the addictive substance rather than true nouishment. A chi deficiency can lead to a range of emotional, social, spiritual, and physical disharmonies.

- Dopamine arouses the pleasures of the sympathetic nervous system. It lifts depression and makes us feel energized and generally happy. Stimulants such as amphetamines and caffeine mimic the dopamine effect.
- **Endorphins and enkephalin** are released as a by-product of stimulation of the PSNS. Endorphins are "the morphine within"; they calm anxiety, elevate mood, and soothe frazzled nerves. When endorphin levels are low, you feel on edge. Sedatives such as tranquilizers mimic the endorphin response and have a calming effect on anxiety.
- **Epinephrine (adrenaline) and norepinephrine** are natural antidepressants. They're triggered by caffeine, alcohol, sugar, and tobacco.
- **Serotonin** contributes to feelings of calmness, better sleep patterns, increased pain resistance, and fewer cravings for carbohydrates. It, too, is a natural antidepressant. Low serotonin levels can cause aggression, depression, food cravings, insomnia, a low pain threshold, and poor temperature regulation by the body. Serotonin levels are particularly affected by both sugar and tobacco.
- **GABA** is a calming neurotransmitter that helps minimize excitatory messages to the brain. GABA works as a muscle relaxant and helps calm anxiety. It also inhibits the desire for alcohol and cocaine. Caffeine, nicotine, alcohol, and other drugs all cause depletion of GABA.

Beating Addictions

No one ever intends to become addicted. But most of us underestimate the power an addictive substance can have, and we overestimate our power of self-control. But just as habits can be acquired, so can they be broken. Others have done it, and you can, too!

Addiction-Free—Naturally teaches you how to replace negative habits with positive ones. In giving up your addiction, you'll learn how to nourish your body, mind, and soul, and how to stay healthy and addiction-free for life.

There's no one method that works for everyone, so *Addiction-Free—Naturally* offers a variety of safe and natural addiction-beating techniques. Their only side effect is better health. Rather than just quitting without any support except willpower, you will now have at your disposal recipes, remedies, and rituals to nourish brain chemistry, stabilize blood sugar levels, correct nutritional deficiencies, and calm the anxieties that keep you craving.

Remember, it took more than a few days for a habit to become your addiction, and it will take more than a few days for you to banish it from your life. The next chapter will introduce you to natural remedies that have benefited others and can be of help to you.

Good luck!

2

On Your
Own Terms

Beating Addictions with
Natural Therapies

This is it. You've made up your mind. You're going to kick this damned addiction for once and for all. You may have tried to quit before, but failed. If so, you're in good company; more than half of all people with addictions try to quit every year, and don't. But never mind that; now I'm going to help you quit for good. How will I do it, you ask? Naturally, I respond—mindfully, conscientiously, safely, positively, spiritually, emotionally, determinedly, bravely, and with all the forces of nature helping you.

There's no doubt about it, kicking an addiction is hard work. It takes willpower, determination, and a whole lotta little pep talks for yourself. But to be successful, most people must do more than simply quit cold turkey. To safely shepherd themselves through the withdrawal period, they must nourish their bodies, ease their anxieties, calm their minds, strengthen their resolve, uplift their spirits, soothe their frazzled nerves, and, above all, remind themselves over and over again of the absolutely compelling and passionate love they have for a healthy, addiction-free life. The natural therapies suggested in this chapter can help. They focus not only on helping you recover from a physical addiction, but on rebuilding a healthy and balanced body, mind, and soul.

Before quitting, really get to know the mechanics of your addiction. Watch yourself in the mirror as you smoke, drink, eat, or so on. Look yourself in the eyes. Be present with the experience. Pay attention to the details of your indulgence. Connect with who you are and what you're doing.

I recently spoke with a woman who told me she ate five doughnuts a day. She usually did this while running up and down the stairs at work, going to get the mail and moving around her office. I suggested that the next day she eat one doughnut, very slowly. Sit down. Do nothing else. Close her eyes. Feel the fat on her tongue. Savor the cheap flavorings in her mouth. Don't read or work; just be with the doughnut. Chew every bite fifty times. Experience mindfulness and presentness as she engaged in addictive behavior. To her surprise, she found the experience distasteful. She didn't want to eat more doughnuts!

Natural Therapies for Beating Addictions

Counseling
Support groups
Prayer
Positive affirmation
Visualization
Journaling
Art therapy
Breathwork
Exercise
Nutrition
Vitamin therapy
Herbs
Homeopathy
Massage and bodywork
Acupressure and acupuncture
Aromatherapy
Flower essences
Light therapy
Color therapy
Gem and crystal therapy

Therapy and Counseling

Simply avoiding the substance you're addicted to is not the entire extent of kicking an addiction. You must also understand *why* you've come to have an addiction. Good counseling or therapy can help you get to the deeper roots of the problem, and can be of great help during the transitional period.

Sometimes a habit gets worse before it improves—perhaps because becoming more aware of it reminds you of doing it. Perhaps the stress of trying to give it up actually makes you need it more. Just persevere. It's only temporary. Keep trying.

Counselors can help you answer questions such as: Why do I feel unable to resist this addiction? Is there anything I can do to overcome this feeling of powerlessness? They can help you reach a state in which you can affirm, I'm not going to let any issues from the past ruin my future. They can allow you to gain and maintain a sense of personal power over the circumstances of your addiction, helping you to acknowledge the issues surrounding your addiction and to find ways of dealing with them. A good counselor can be your best friend both in making the decision to kick your addiction and in staying addiction-free.

Support Groups

Alcoholics Anonymous (AA) was founded in 1935 by Bill Wilson, a stockbroker, and Bob Smith, a physician, both alcoholics who helped each other get sober and who brought their message to others. AA has become a tremendously powerful and successful support group that has helped millions of alcoholics all around the world give up drinking and recover healthy, positive lives. AA created the mold for many of the addiction-related support groups that exist today.

Support groups offer the soul-warming support and guidance of others who have been there. Many people feel more comfortable talking to others who are in the same situation as they are, who face the same challenges and suffer from the same pain, and support groups offer this open, empathetic atmosphere. They can help you talk through emotional tangles related to your addiction, and they can even give you someone to call during difficult times who can give you comfort and help you stay focused on being addiction-free.

I highly recommend that people struggling to give up an addiction join a support group. Look in the yellow pages of your phone book or on the Internet to find a group that meets in your location.

The Power of Prayer

Prayer is a powerful tool. It's good for body, mind, and spirit, and it's free. So let go and let God/dess help you. You have a direct line to that higher, greater-than-ourselves power. Use it. Ask for divine help. It is available.

If you don't have any particular religious beliefs and are uncomfortable praying to a higher power, you can use a meditative type of prayer. Simply sit quietly and clear your mind of thoughts. Feel warmth and nourishment being received from the center of the Youniverse. Join with this holy energy, asking for help in being free of addiction.

Prayer gets easier with practice. It can even become a ritual practiced during many everyday activities, such as walking, bathing, and simply being.

> Alcoholics who practice transcendental meditation report a steady decline in alcohol use as well as a 90 percent sobriety record after two years.

Positive Affirmations

So long as we see ourselves as stuck and addicted, we will be. If we see ourselves as wonderful, healthy, love-worthy beings, we have no need for addictions.

Affirmations are prepared positive thoughts that you repeat to yourself, out loud, over and over again. If you say something often enough, eventually your mind begins to believe it. By repeating a positive affirmation, you reprogram your thought patterns in a positive direction. When you convince your mind that you are a person for whom addiction holds no attraction, it begins to become true. Many studies—and millions of people—have proven the efficacy of positive affirmations.

Say your affirmations upon rising in the morning, during quiet periods of the day, and before drifting off to sleep. Affirmations work even better if you say them standing in front of a mirror, making eye contact with yourself, repeating the words forcefully as if trying to convince this person before you.

Louise Hay, author of *Heal Your Body*, says that addictions are "running from the self. Fear. Not knowing how to love the self." Affirmations you might choose to reverse these feelings include:

- I now discover how wonderful I am. I choose to love and enjoy myself.
- I live in the now. Each moment is new. I choose to see my self-worth. I love and approve of myself.

Whenever faced with temptation, you can repeat affirmations such as:

- I am strong. I am getting better. I am able to resist.
- I release the need to indulge in _____ (coffee, cigarettes, alcohol, et cetera).

Visualization

Visualization is another method of reprogramming your mind. In a quiet, almost meditative state, visualize yourself as the addiction-free person you want to be, or visualize different symbolic methods of letting go of your addiction.

For example, imagine that you are holding on to a balloon string; at the base of the balloon is a basket. Into that basket put all the negative things in your life—your addiction, lack of love, rejection, guilt, and so on. Lift your hand and visualize letting go of the balloon.

Or visualize yourself getting through those moments or emotions in which you're most likely to indulge in your addiction with grace, humor, and goodwill—and without the crutch of your addiction.

In moments of stress you can practice visualization to help you relax. For example, visualize a clear bubble surrounding you that expands as you inhale and contracts as you exhale. Imagine the most beautiful place possible—a beach, forest, cottage—whatever best comforts and calms you. Create as much detail as possible. Then bring this safe place inside your bubble. The more you practice this visualization, the easier it will become, and in time you'll be able to call it up in an instant, whenever you start to feel stressed or anxious.

There are many possible forms of visualization. If you can't find one that works for you, sample some of the commercial recordings of guided visualizations that are available in most bookstores. (See the resource section on page 232 for suggestions.) You can also record your own visualization session on a tape and play it back to yourself. Or find a therapist who works with guided visualization, and work together with him or her on building one that's right for you.

Ayurvedic medicine combines chakra consciousness with color for a powerful healing visualization. Chakras are the seven energy centers in the body that correspond to states of consciousness and physical health. When a chakra becomes blocked, proper functioning in this area is affected. For example, a person with a chakra blockage in the solar plexus may have difficulty assimilating food, have bloating or gas, or experience stomach pain. Sending healing energy and acknowledgment to each chakra can help clear such blockages.

Preparing for Visualization

Find a comfortable, quiet location. Lie down or sit in a comfortable position. If it's cold, cover up with a blanket. Close your eyes. Breathe deeply. Focus on the in and out of your breath. Feel your lungs expand and contract, the breath moving in your nostrils, and the coolness of air passing through your throat. Try to block out any other thoughts. Tell yourself that you're taking a time-out. In ten minutes—or five, or twenty, or for however long you practice visualization—you will return to these thoughts, but for just these few precious minutes you're putting them aside. When you feel relaxed, begin the visualization.

The chakras each correspond to a particular color. If you visualize sending the appropriate healing color to a chakra, you turn it on, clearing blockages and activating its energy. Close your eyes and mentally feel out each chakra. Then begin visualizing each chakra surrounded by and suffused with its corresponding color. Keep up each chakra visualization for about a minute, then move on to the next.

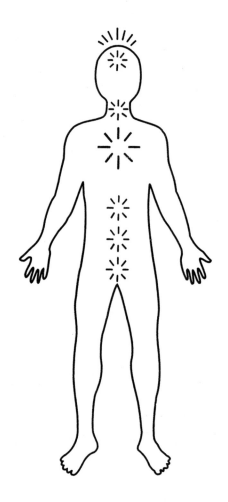

Chakra	Color
Base of the spine	Red
Genitals	Orange
Navel or solar plexus	Yellow
Heart	Green
Throat	Blue
Third eye, or the point between the brows	Indigo
Top of the head, or crown chakra	Indigo

Journaling to Overcome Addiction

Overcoming addiction can be an experience of really getting to know your inner self. Creativity is an excellent means of acknowledging and expressing inner emotions, and journal writing is a great place to begin. Buy yourself a journal and allow this to become a place where you can bare your soul in private. Write private poetry about your struggle with addiction. Explore your angst.

Try writing to your habit with your right hand, describing how it affects you. Then, with your left hand, have your addiction "write back to you." What does it want from you? Why is it with you?

Good questions to ponder in your writings include:

- How does this addiction serve me?
- What issues does this addiction keep me from having to deal with?
- What is addiction preventing me from having to do? Get a job? Have a relationship? Be social, sexual, or physical?
- What was going on in my life in the year or two prior to the addiction?
- What do I want life to look like one year from now? Five years from now? Ten years from now? What do I need to do to get there?
- What can I learn from this experience?
- If I persist in this habit, what are the three worst possible consequences?
- What important gains are there if I give up this habit?
- Why can't I just let go of this addiction?
- How would I live life if no more _____ (cigarettes, alcohol, sugar, et cetera) existed?

A journal can become a tracking system for your addiction, allowing you to pinpoint the emotions and situations that trigger it. In your journal note how you feel both before and after you indulge in your addiction. Write down the time of day for each incident, what was going on around you, what you were thinking about, and how you felt. Notice when you are most at risk and what triggers the habit—the clues, buzzwords, emotions. Once you can identify these triggers, you can learn to avoid or overcome them.

Art Therapy

"Art is toxic discharge," said a wise teacher of mine, Michael Tierra. Working with your hands helps improve your self-esteem and gives you a new focus for an addiction-free life. Learn to paint, draw, knit, crochet, carve, build, weld, make jewelry, macramé, sculpt, garden. Play an instrument. Write a song. It's never too late to take lessons or take up again a craft or hobby you enjoyed as a youth.

Draw pictures of your addiction. A monkey on your back? A dog biting your butt? Putting it on paper helps get it out of your system.

Breathwork for Overcoming Addiction

Breathing is the one automatic biological activity that can be completely controlled. And how we breathe affects our health and consciousness. Generally speaking, deep breathing—pulling the air all the way down into the belly—can both calm and energize us. In times of stress—say, for example, when an addiction craving strikes—breathing exercises can help relax the mind and ease tension. Here are several deep-breathing techniques that you can experiment with:

- **Deep relaxation breath.** Lie on the floor with a pillow below your knees. Place your hands over your stomach, palms down, with your fingers gently laced just above your navel. Breathe in through your nostrils to a count of three, feeling your abdomen push the fingers up toward the ceiling. Exhale to a count of five as your fingers and abdomen move toward the floor. Repeat ten times.
- **The complete breath.** Lie in a quiet place with your arms at your sides, palms down. Close your eyes and slowly inhale through your nostrils, feeling your abdomen expand, then your

rib cage, and finally your upper chest. Hold for a few seconds. Breathe out slowly while drawing in your abdomen and relaxing the chest and rib cage. Then inhale again, slowly raising your arms, in synchronization with your breath, above and behind your head until the back of each hand touches the floor. Keep each arm as straight as possible as you stretch. Hold for ten seconds. As you slowly exhale, bring your arms back to your sides. Repeat the entire procedure several times.

- **Alternate-nostril breathing.** This breathwork technique helps bring more air into the lungs and move accumulated pollutants. It's quite simple and can be practiced anywhere. First breathe in through both nasal passages. Then close one nostril with a finger and exhale through the remaining open passage. Breathe in and out through that open side, keeping the other nostril closed. Repeat on the other side.

Deep, steady breathing can be a surprisingly effective deterrent to addiction. During the day, check in with yourself. Pay attention to your breathing. Make a conscious effort to breathe deep the breath of life.

The Lean, Mean, Addiction-Fighting Machine

Exercise improves the health of the body, mind, and spirit. Exercise boosts circulation, moves blockages in the body, improves digestion, lifts depression, and relieves anxiety. It also enhances the brain chemicals endorphins and enkephalin, which can relieve pain and elevate mood.

There are many different kinds of exercise that are good for both body and soul. Dance helps you "go with the flow." Put on music from a time you associate with safety and happiness and dance to your heart's delight. Walking lets you introduce yourself to the neighbors. Hiking brings you in contact with the healing power of nature. Biking allows you to race like the wind. Kickboxing and martial arts classes help you feel strong and independent. Do whatever it is that you enjoy. The important thing is to get out there!

Yoga

Yoga is an extremely effective form of ritualized healing exercise. In a study conducted by the Yoga Biomedical Trust of London, of 219 tobacco smokers who started practicing yoga, 74 percent felt it helped them in overcoming addiction.

Early in your process of recovering from any addiction, choose low-impact exercises such as yoga, tai chi, or simple stretching.

Specific yoga poses for overcoming addiction are those that aid in clearing substances from the liver. Examples include the Locust, the Shoulder Stand, the Plow, and the Fish Pose. I highly recommend that you join a yoga class in your area; ask the instructor to include these poses, or other liver-cleansing poses, in the routines that he or she teaches.

Nutrition

Keeping your blood sugar on a normal level, correcting nutritional deficiencies, and cleansing the body are the nutritional keys to overcoming addictions. In general, eat a high-fiber diet, which promotes good elimination, and drink plenty of fluids, especially pure water. Choose foods that are as unprocessed, chemical-free, and close to their natural state as possible. Go for nourishing food that tastes good.

Most addictions arise from a sugar dependency. In addition to being an addiction itself, sugar dependency can contribute to many other addictions. To keep your blood sugar level steady, eat small, frequent meals. Cut out sugary snacks, which can cause your blood sugar to swing wildly between high and low levels. If you need a sweetener, use brown rice syrup or honey.

Refined carbohydrates are another form of simple sugar that should be eliminated from your diet. They include bread, pancakes, waffles, bagels, pasta—just about anything made with white flour. Instead, eat more whole grains such as brown rice, buckwheat, millet, and barley to keep your blood sugar on an even keel. Oatmeal is used in Ayurvedic medicine to treat opium addiction.

Miso is also good for stabilizing blood sugar levels. When you're feeling a late-afternoon crash and start craving some sugar, mix a bit of miso in with some warm water and drink. This pick-me-up broth will quell your craving and bring your blood sugar level back to a normal condition.

To prevent intense addiction cravings, consume small amounts of protein every couple of hours. Good protein sources include fish, poultry, legumes, tofu, tempeh, nuts, seeds, eggs, and good-quality cheese. Fish is high in amino acids and very supportive to brain chemistry. Nuts and seeds such as almonds, sesame seeds, sunflower seeds, and pumpkin seeds are good protein sources that also contain essential fatty acids, which can reduce withdrawal symptoms, mini-minimize cravings, and help you feel more calm and alert. Black soybeans are especially tonifying for depleted adrenal glands and kidneys. Fava and lima beans help the body produce dopamine, which can lift depression and enhance feelings of well-being.

Eat plenty of foods that help the liver cleanse itself, including apples, artichokes, beets, burdock root, carrots, celery, daikon radish, green leafy vegetables (dandelion greens, kale, collards, and watercress), and sweet potatoes.

Make sea vegetables such as dulse, kelp, kombu, nori, and wakame a regular part of your diet. They help nourish the thyroid gland and endocrine system, and they improve metabolism, help you maintain normal weight, and provide a multitude of trace minerals.

Superfoods such as barley grass juice, wheat grass juice, blue-green algae, spirulina, and chlorella are also important elements of a rebuilding diet. They are highly nutritive, rich in chlorophyll and amino acids, and easy to digest.

Do your best to drink plenty of pure water. Juice made from carrots, beets, celery, string beans, or any dark green leafy vegetable such as spinach, watercress, or wheat grass can also be used to help cleanse the system. Note, however, that fruit and vegetable juices are very high in sugars and lacking in fiber. Dilute them by half with water to avoid overstimulating the pancreas.

An adequate amount of dietary fat helps nourish and lubricate a frazzled nervous system. It also aids in serotonin production, which calms the mind and enhances the feeling of well-being. Olive, flaxseed, and hempseed oils are good sources. Organic, unsweetened yogurt is also very nourishing for the nerves and helps repair the digestive system.

> **Foods for Fighting Alcoholism**
>
> Kohlrabi and mung bean sprouts aid in detoxification from alcohol. Also try winter melon, a traditional Chinese medicine remedy for alcoholism. You may be able to find it in an Asian foods market.

Use small amounts of warming spices such as cardamom, cinnamon, cloves, cumin, ginger, mustard seeds, and pepper as condiments to help improve circulation and digestion.

Create a feeling of security by eating warming soups and stews and lightly cooked vegetables. These warm, pleasant-tasting foods stimulate endorphin production, which helps the body relax and produces a sense of well-being.

Though warm foods should be the dietary emphasis for someone struggling to give up an addiction, small amounts of raw fruits can also be helpful. Fruits are cleansing and supply the body with natural sugars and nutrients. Many fruits can assist you in giving up an addiction:

- **Apples** lubricate the lungs and help relieve intoxication. They're high in pectin, which binds with toxins such as tobacco smoke and carries them out of the body.
- **Pears**, a close relative of apples, are used in traditional Chinese medicine to treat alcoholism.
- **Berries** help clean the blood and liver.
- **Figs** contain natural sugars that are also rich in antioxidants and have a cleansing effect.
- **Bananas** aid in detoxification, and their natural sugars help relieve cravings during withdrawal. In traditional Chinese medicine a tea of organic banana peel is recommended to relieve hangovers and alcoholism. Practitioners of folk medicine in Hawaii suggest banana, papaya, and pineapple to overcome the desire to consume alcohol and tobacco.

Supplement Therapy for Addiction

It's imperative to nourish the body and provide it with necessary nutrients to help calm anxiety, lessen cravings, and give support during times of stress. Recovering addicts who use supplements stay in treatment longer and generally do better than those who don't.

Vitamins and Minerals

Vitamin and mineral supplements are readily available at any grocery store, and they can do wonders for someone struggling to give up an addiction.

- **Vitamin A** is an antioxidant that strengthens resistance to infections and makes mucous membranes less permeable to infection. Take 5,000 to 25,000 international units (IU) once daily. Or take 20,000 to 40,000 milligrams of beta-carotene daily. Beta-carotene is converted to vitamin A in the body.
- **B-complex vitamins** are calming and nourishing to the nerves. They can help balance moods, diminish withdrawal symptoms, stabilize fluctations in energy, and aid in liver regeneration. B-complex vitamins can also reduce neuritis and pellagra, both common in alcohol abuse. Take 25 to 100 milligrams of a B-complex supplement every day.

The B Vitamins

- **Vitamin B1 (thiamin)** is depleted by the use of coffee, alcohol, sugar, and tobacco. It's needed for normal nerve conduction; a deficiency can contribute to feelings of fear and anxiety.
- **Vitamin B2** is often deficient as a result of alcohol consumption.
- **Vitamin B3 (niacin)** is also commonly deficient as a result of alcohol consumption. Niacin helps regulate blood sugar levels and minimizes detoxification reactions.
- **Vitamin B6** improves energy and assists metabolism.
- **Vitamin B12** is often deficient in smokers and alcoholics.
- **Choline** is a member of the B-complex family that helps in breaking down fats in the liver and in maintaining healthy kidneys.
- **Folic acid** deficiency is common in smokers, alcoholics, and those who use barbiturates.

- **Vitamin C** is one of the most essential nutrients for detoxifying from addictions. It can reduce cravings and helps protect the body against acetaldehyde. Vitamin C also helps detoxify the liver and blood and nourishes the adrenal glands. Take 1,000 milligrams every two to four hours during withdrawal until cravings have passed. Then decrease the amount to twice daily. Buffered vitamin C is easiest on the stomach.
- **Vitamin E** is an antioxidant and thus protects against free-radical damage to the body's cells. It also can help repair damaged liver function. Take 200 to 800 international units per day.
- **Calcium** aids in neurotransmitter release and heartbeat regulation. It calms the nervous system and promotes good sleep and rest. Take 800 to 1,500 milligrams daily.
- **Magnesium** helps stabilize blood sugar levels, relieves spasms, relaxes muscles, and calms nerves. It decreases extreme nerve sensitivity and helps calm anxiety and stress. Take 400 to 750 milligrams daily.
- **Potassium** is essential for healthy nervous system function. Alcohol, sugar, and coffee all deplete the body of potassium. Take 100 to 300 milligrams daily.
- **Zinc** ensures proper immune function and promotes healing. It also helps in maintenance of taste and smell senses and normalizes appetite. Alcoholics in particular are usually deficient in zinc. Take 30 to 60 milligrams of chelated zinc every day.
- **Selenium** is an antioxidant that helps prevent free-radical damage, including premature aging. It helps protect the liver from alcohol-induced liver disease as well as against damage from tobacco smoke. Take 200 to 300 micrograms daily.
- **Iron** helps transport oxygen from the lungs to the body's tissues. A deficiency in iron can contribute to low energy and anemia. Take 10 to 30 milligrams daily.
- **Chromium** is an essential nutrient for stabilizing blood sugar levels. It also helps reduce cravings. Take 200 to 1,000 micrograms daily.

Essential Fatty Acids

Essential fatty acids (EFAs) keep brain and nerve function stable, allowing you to feel generally calmer and more alert and helping you deal with stress. An EFA deficiency can aggravate addictions and their behavioral cohorts: attention deficit disorder, anxiety, and depression. It may be that the opposite is also true; in the 1950s researcher Johanna Budwig suggested that essential fatty acids could treat a wide range of addictive behavior. And it's been proven that supplementing with EFAs can reduce withdrawal symptoms and minimize cravings.

> Both calcium and magnesium are helpful in giving the nervous system the support it will need when giving up an addiction.

Hempseed and flaxseed oils are excellent sources of EFAs, and they also help restore normal hormonal function. Take 1 to 3 tablespoons or 2 to 6 capsules daily.

Evening primrose oil is another good source of EFAs. It also encourages healing of liver damage and can ease the withdrawal from alcohol. Take 1 or 2 capsules three times daily.

Amino Acids

Amino acids are another important group of supplements that can help you beat an addiction. They are sometimes available in combinations specially designed to support brain function.

Caution: If you have lupus or are taking methadone, consult with your physician before taking amino acid supplements.

- **DL-phenylalanine** is an amino acid essential for the formation of several neurotransmitters, including dopamine, epinephrine, and norepinephrine. DL-phenylalanine helps reduce physical pain and depression by both stimulating production of endorphins and inhibiting their breakdown. Take 500 to 1,500 milligrams daily. *Caution:* Do not use DL-phenylalanine if you suffer from phenylketonuria, melanoma, migraines, or hepatic cirrhosis.
- **Glutathione** is a combination of three amino acids: cysteine, glutamate, and glycine. It's a powerful antioxidant and aids in

liver detoxification. Glutathione also enables the liver to break down dangerous compounds and excrete them through the bile. Take 250 to 500 milligrams daily.

- **5 hydroxytryptophan (HTP)** elevates natural serotonin levels and can relieve depression, anxiety, obsessive-compulsive disorder, and mood swings; improve sleep; and reduce cravings for sweets, drugs, and alcohol. Take 100 milligrams two to three times daily.

- **L-cysteine** aids in detoxification, nourishes the blood, and promotes tissue generation. It protects the brain and liver from damage by alcohol and cigarette consumption and reduces emphysema in smokers. Take 250 to 500 milligrams daily.

- **L-glutamine** is an amino acid that helps reduce cravings and stabilize blood sugar levels by providing ready glucose fuel to the brain. Studies have shown that rats fed glutamine voluntarily reduce their alcohol consumption. L-glutamine also improves mental alertness and helps in the production of GABA (see page 12). Take 250 to 1,000 milligrams daily. To stop intense cravings, open a capsule and let the contents dissolve on your tongue.

- **Taurine** clears toxins from the liver, protects the brain from chemical damage, and stabilizes brain function. It can also help stop tremors associated with withdrawal. Take 250 to 500 milligrams once or twice daily.

- **Tyrosine** helps the body make dopamine and norepinephrine, which work together to elevate mood, ease anxiety, and make you feel happy. It also regulates chi, cleanses the liver, improves memory, and relieves stress, anxiety, and depression. Tyrosine is especially helpful in beating addictions to chocolate and alcohol. Take 100 milligrams daily.

Other Supplements

A variety of other supplements can also be helpful for those struggling to give up an addiction. Most can be found in natural foods stores or supplement shops.

- **Acidophilus.** The intestinal flora in substance abusers is usually greatly imbalanced and can contribute to malabsorption of food and increased allergies. Acidophilus rebalances the digestive tract and inhibits replication of unfriendly yeasts and microorganisms. Take 2 capsules three times daily.
- **Adrenal.** Adrenal glands tend to be exhausted after long-term substance abuse. Taking raw adrenal can help build strength when the body is depleted and exhausted. Take 25 to 50 milligrams daily.
- **Chlorophyll,** the life energy of plants, is extremely purifying and rejuvenating. Take 1 to 3 capsules daily.
- **Coenzyme Q-10** is an antioxidant that aids in the production of ATP (adenosine triphosphate), an important source of energy for the body. Take 50 to 150 milligrams daily.
- **DHA.** A deficiency in DHA (docosahexaenoic acid) can contribute to depression, aggression, and impulsive behavior. Take 1,200 milligrams three times daily.
- **GABA** (gamma-aminobutyric acid) is a calming neurotransmitter that helps minimize excitatory messages to the brain. GABA works as a muscle relaxant and helps calm anxiety. It also inhibits the desire for alcohol and cocaine. Caffeine, nicotine, drugs, and alcohol all cause depletion of GABA. Take 750 milligrams daily.
- **Lecithin** helps rebuild tissue damaged by substance abuse. Take 1 to 3 tablespoons or 2 to 6 capsules daily.
- **Lipoic acid** is an antioxidant and aids in the conversion of carbohydrates to energy. Take 20 to 50 milligrams daily.
- **Pancreatic enzymes** help the body absorb nutrients from food. Take 400 to 500 milligrams three times daily.
- **SAMe** (s-adenosyl-methionine) is composed of the amino acid methionine and ATP. It aids in the manufacture of many brain chemicals, including serotonin, dopamine, and phosphatidylcholine. SAMe helps relieve depression and liver disorders. Take 200 milligrams four times daily. *Caution:* If you suffer from bipolar depression, consult with your physician before using SAMe.

Herbs for Addiction

Herbs have been used as medicine and food for thousands of years by millions of people with positive results. They can be made up into teas, capsules, or tinctures (see chapter 11), or they can be added fresh to your breakfast, lunch, or dinner. Herbs useful for those struggling to give up an addiction are described over the following pages.

Those with alcohol-abuse issues should avoid any tinctures made with alcohol. Consider instead using teas, capsules, vinegar tinctures, or glycerites.

As herbal medicine has grown in popularity, some herbs have been overharvested from the wild. If you're considering using a plant that's a threatened or endangered species, be sure to purchase supplies that were grown commercially—and organically!—and avoid those that were wildcrafted. Better yet, learn to cultivate your own supplies.

Trained herbalists can be very helpful in creating an herbal-based wellness regimen that can help you kick your addiction. For recommendations for herbalists in your area, contact the American Herbalists Guild (see the resources section).

When the plant part used is described as "herb," that means all of a plant's aerial parts: the leaves, flowers, and stem.

Alfalfa

Latin name: *Medicago sativa*

Family: Fabaceae

Parts used: Leaves and flowers

Usage: Alfalfa is useful for those giving up alcohol, tobacco, or any drug. It's considered nutritive and tonic. It relieves fatigue, helps remove drug residue from the body, and aids the body in absorbing nutrients from food. Alfalfa can even be used as a remedy for jaundice.

Dosage: 1 cup of tea three times daily; 2 to 3 capsules three times daily

Energetics: Salty, neutral, moist

Concerns: Those with lupus and rheumatoid arthritis should avoid alfalfa sprouts, although the leaves and flowers are perfectly safe for use.

Aloe Vera

Latin name: *Aloe ferox, A. perryi, A. vera*
Family: Aloaceae
Part used: Gel from leaf
Usage: Aloe has cholagogue, demulcent, hepatic, rejuvenative, and vulnerary properties. It soothes lungs irritated from cigarette smoke and helps balance liver function.
Dosage: 1 shot glass ten minutes before meals three times daily
Energetics: Bitter, cool, moist
Concerns: Avoid internal use during pregnancy. Aloe should not be used by those suffering from abdominal pain; if abdominal pain occurs, discontinue use.

Amla

Also known as: Emblic, ambal
Latin name: *Phyllanthus emblica*
Family: Euphorbiaceae
Part used: Fruit
Usage: Amla serves as a laxative, a nutritive, and a stomach tonic. It's specific to food addiction. It increases lean body mass while reducing fat.
Dosage: 1 cup of tea three times daily; 30 to 40 drops of tincture three times daily
Energetics: Sour, sweet, cool
Concerns: Avoid in cases of acute diarrhea and dysentery.

Angelica

Also known as: Bai zhi
Latin name: *Angelica archangelica, A. atropurpea*
Family: Apiaceae
Part Used: Roots
Usage: Angelica is a nervine and a tonic. Taken as a tea or in capsule form, it helps create a distaste for alcohol.
Dosage: 1 cup of tea three times daily; 40 to 60 drops of tincture three times daily
Energetics: Sweet, pungent, warm, dry

Concerns: Use only the dried root. Angelica should not be used by diabetics or pregnant women. Large doses can affect blood pressure, nerves, and respiration. It can cause photosensitivity in some people.

Aniseed

Also known as: Huei-hsiang
Latin name: *Pimpinella anisum*
Family: Apiaceae
Part used: Seeds
Usage: Aniseed is antispasmodic and tonic. It elevates blood sugar levels naturally, reducing sugar-based cravings for drugs and alcohol. It also builds chi and energy.
Dosage: 1 cup of tea three times daily; 40 to 60 drops of tincture three times daily
Energetics: Sweet, pungent, warm
Concerns: Avoid therapeutic dosages during pregnancy unless directed by your health professional.

Ashwagandha

Also known as: Winter cherry
Latin name: *Withania somnifera*
Family: Solanaceae
Part used: Roots
Usage: Ashwagandha functions as an adaptogen, antispasmodic, nerve restorative, nutritive, rejuvenative, sedative, and tonic. It's especially helpful for treating drug and alcohol addictions, and it makes a wonderful tonic for those who work excessively. Ashwagandha lifts the spirits, relieves depression, helps rebuild the nervous system, and can be used to treat anxiety, memory loss, mental fatigue, stress, and tremors. In Ayurvedic medicine ashwagandha is specific for Vata types with addictions.
Dosage: 1 cup of tea three times daily; 30 to 40 drops of tincture three times daily
Energetics: Bitter, sweet, warm
Concerns: Avoid during pregnancy. Do not take in combination with barbiturates, because it may increase barbiturates' potency.

Asparagus

Also known as: Tian men dong, Shatavari (Sanskrit)

Latin name: *Asparagus officinalis, A. racemosus, A. cochinchinensis*

Family: Liliaceae

Parts used: Roots, rhizomes

Usage: Asparagus is a nutritive, rejuvenative, kidney tonic, and sedative. It helps balance emotions, calms irritability and oversensitivity, and improves memory. Use during convalescence.

Dosage: 1 cup of tea three times daily; 30 to 40 drops of tincture
three times daily

Energetics: Bitter, sweet, moist, cool

Concerns: Safe when used appropriately.

Astragalus

Also known as: Huang chi

Latin name: *Astragalus membranaceus, A. mongholicus*

Family: Fabaceae

Part used: Roots

Usage: Astragalus is an adaptogen, adrenal tonic, and blood, lung,
and chi tonic. It improves nutrient assimilation and increases
energy. Astragalus also inhibits free-radical formation, thus helping restore immune system function.

Dosage: 1 cup of tea three times daily; 30 to 60 drops of tincture
three times daily

Energetics: Sweet, warm

Concerns: If you're using astragalus during an acute infection, combine
it with diaphoretic herbs. Otherwise it's safe when used appropriately.

Atractylodes

Also known as: Bai zhu

Latin name: *Atractylodes alba, A. lancea, A. macrocephala*

Family: Asteraceae

Part used: Rhizomes

Usage: Atractylodes functions as a restorative and a chi and liver
tonic. It improves digestion, counteracts hypoglycemia, and increases energy.

Dosage: ½ cup of tea three times daily; 20 drops of tincture three times daily

Energetics: Bitter, sweet, warm

Concerns: Atractylodes is safe when used appropriately, as described here. In larger doses it can aggravate bleeding ulcers and dehydration.

Barberry

Also known as: Oregon grape root, Daruharidra (Sanskrit)

Latin name: *Berberis aquifolium, Mahonia nervosa, M. repens*

Family: Berberidaceae

Parts used: Roots, root bark

Usage: Barberry is an alterative, anti-inflammatory, cholagogue, and liver tonic. It helps clear negative emotions from the liver and heat from the lungs, which can be especially helpful for smokers.

Dosage: ½ to 1 cup of tea three times daily; 10 to 20 drops of tincture three times daily

Energetics: Bitter, cold

Concerns: Use only the dried plant, because the fresh plant can cause nausea and be purgative. Avoid during pregnancy and in cases of hyperthyroid. Barberry is at risk of becoming endangered in the wild, so do not use wildcrafted supplies.

Basil

Also known as: Lui le, Tulsi (Sanskrit)

Latin name: *Ocimum basilicum*

Family: Lamiaceae

Part used: Herb

Usage: Basil not only tastes great but also functions as an antidepressant, antispasmodic, circulatory stimulant, digestive tonic, nervine, and sedative. It lifts the spirits from depression and calms anxiety. Use for alcoholism, drug overdose, and to calm the mind and body during withdrawal.

Dosage: 1 cup of tea three times daily; 10 to 30 drops of tincture three times daily

Energetics: Pungent, warm, dry

Concerns: Young children and pregnant women should avoid therapeutic dosages (anything more than what you use to season your food) during pregnancy. Basil should not be used for extended periods at large doses.

Bayberry

Also known as: Wax myrtle, Katphala (Sanskrit)
Latin name: *Myrica cerifera, M. pensylvanica*
Family: Myricaceae
Parts used: Roots, bark
Usage: Bayberry functions as an alterative, antispasmodic, circulatory stimulant, expectorant, and stimulant. In particular, it encourages healing of the mucous membranes. It's especially useful for those trying to quit smoking.
Dosage: 1/4 cup of tea three times daily; 10 to 30 drops of tincture three times daily
Energetics: Pungent, warm
Concerns: Avoid during pregnancy and in cases of hot conditions such as fever, high blood pressure, and inflammation. Large doses may be emetic.

Blue Vervain

Also known as: Ma bian cao
Latin name: *Verbena officinalis*
Family: Verbenaceae
Part used: Herb
Usage: Blue vervain improves liver function and acts as a nerve restorative. It's an antispasmodic, cardiotonic, cholagogue, expectorant, hepato-stimulant, nervine, and sedative. It can be used to treat a variety of conditions, including anxiety, cirrhosis, depression, headache, hepatitis, hysteria, insomnia, nervousness, pain, and stress.
Dosage: 1/2 cup of tea three times daily; 10 to 20 drops of tincture three times daily
Energetics: Pungent, bitter, cold
Concerns: Avoid during pregnancy, except during labor and as prescribed by your health care practitioner. Large amounts may be emetic.

Bupleurum

Also known as: Chinese thoroughwax, hare's ear root, Chai hu

Latin name: *Bupleurum falcatum, B. chinense, B. scorzoneraefolium*

Family: Apiaceae

Part used: Roots

Usage: Bupleurum is a harmonizing herb often called for in traditional Chinese medicine and Ayurvedic medicine. It functions as an alterative, chi tonic, choleretic, diaphoretic, hepato-protectant, muscle relaxant, and tonic. It moves liver stagnation, improves adrenal function, and helps clear anger, depression, grief, moodiness, stress, and pain. It's especially helpful in reducing the emotional factors associated with addiction.

Dosage: ½ cup of tea three times daily; 30 to 40 drops of tincture three times daily

Energetics: Pungent, bitter, cool

Concerns: Avoid in cases of hot conditions such as fever, high blood pressure, and inflammation. Long-term use may cause dizziness. Otherwise it's safe when used appropriately.

Burdock

Also known as: Bardane, clotburr, gypsy rhubarb, gobo, Wu shih, Niu bang (seeds)

Latin name: *Arctium lappa*

Family: Asteraceae

Parts used: Roots, seeds

Usage: Burdock has alterative, choleretic, demulcent, nutritive, and rejuvenative properties. It cleanses the liver and blood of drug residues and can be used to calm both anger and pain. It also improves the function of all the organs of elimination and improves the metabolism of fats, which makes it particularly useful for those trying to give up food addictions.

Dosage: 1 cup of tea three times daily; 10 to 30 drops of tincture three times daily

Energetics: Bitter, cool, dry

Concerns: Safe when used appropriately. However, women in the first trimester of pregnancy should avoid using the seeds.

Calamus

Also known as: Sweet flag, singer's root, sweet sedge, Shi chang pu, Vacha (Sanskrit)

Latin name: *Acorus calamus*

Family: Araceae

Part used: Rhizomes

Usage: Calamus is analgesic, antispasmodic, rejuvenative, sedative, stimulant, and tonic. It's a great tonic for the psyche: it clears the mind, soothes the nervous system, helps restore mental faculties, calms hysteria, eases depression, and enhances perception. Calamus is used in Ayurvedic medicine to reduce the emotional need for drugs. When combined with tobacco, calamus causes nausea, so it's sometimes chewed or smoked as a deterrent to smoking.

Dosage: ½ cup of tea three times daily; 5 to 30 drops of tincture three times daily

Energetics: Bitter, pungent, warm, dry

Concerns: Use only American varieties of calamus. Avoid during pregnancy. Otherwise it's safe when used appropriately. Calamus is considered at risk of becoming endangered in the wild, so don't use wildcrafted supplies.

California Poppy

Latin name: *Eschscholzia californica*

Family: Papaveraceae

Parts used: Roots, herb

Usage: California poppy functions as an analgesic, anodyne, antispasmodic, hypnotic, nervine, sedative, and soporific. It calms the spirit, anxiety, and restlessness. Use when giving up alcohol, tobacco, or prescription drugs.

Dosage: 1 cup of tea three times daily; 20 to 40 drops of tincture three times daily

Energetics: Bitter, cool

Concerns: Avoid in cases of depression. California poppy is not addictive, as some of its more famous poppy cousins are, but excessive use may cause you to feel somewhat hungover in the morning. Do not combine with MAO-inhibiting drugs.

Cardamom

Also known as: Grains of paradise, Bai dou kou, Ela (Sanskrit)

Latin name: *Elettaria cardamomum*

Family: Zingiberaceae

Part used: Seeds

Usage: Cardamom is an antispasmodic, aromatic, carminative, cerebral stimulant, expectorant, thermogenic, and tonic, and it's a great spice to keep in your cabinet. It helps lift depression, relieve fatigue, build chi, and improve circulation to the digestive system.

Dosage: 1 cup of tea three times daily; 10 to 20 drops of tincture three times daily

Energetics: Pungent, bitter, sweet, warm, dry

Concerns: Safe when used appropriately.

Catnip

Also known as: Catmint, Chi hsueh tsao

Latin name: *Nepeta cataria*

Family: Lamiaceae

Part used: Herb

Usage: Plant some in your yard for both you and your feline friends! In humans catnip functions as an antispasmodic, nervine, sedative, and tonic. It can be used to ease anxiety, irritability, nervousness, and restlessness. It's especially helpful for those giving up tobacco.

Dosage: 1 cup of tea two or three times daily; 20 to 40 drops of tincture three times daily

Energetics: Pungent, bitter, cool, dry

Concerns: Avoid during pregnancy.

Cayenne Pepper

Also known as: African pepper, bird pepper, chili pepper, Marichiphalam (Sanskrit)

Latin name: *Capsicum frutescens, C. annuum*

Family: Solanaceae

Part used: Fruit

Usage: Cayenne is alterative, antioxidant, diaphoretic, expectorant, stimulant, thermogenic—and hot! It improves circulation, moves obstructions of chi, and warms chills. It's especially helpful for those struggling to give up addictions to alcohol and drugs.

Dosage: 1 capsule three times daily; 5 to 15 drops of tincture three times daily

Energetics: Pungent, hot, dry

Concerns: Keep away from the eyes and mucous membranes. Wash your hands after contact with the herb. Avoid therapeutic dosages when you're pregnant or nursing. Large amounts can irritate the gastrointestinal tract and kidneys.

Celery

Latin name: *Apium graveolens*
Family: Apiaceae
Part used: Seeds
Usage: Celery seed is an alterative, nervine, sedative, tonic, and urinary antiseptic. It helps soothe the nerves and relieve pain, and it can be used to counter alcohol, caffeine, and tobacco addictions.
Dosage: 1 cup of tea three times daily; 20 to 40 drops of tincture three times daily
Energetics: Bitter, sweet, cool, moist
Concerns: Large amounts may increase photosensitivity. Pregnant women and those with kidney disorders should avoid large doses.

Centaury

Also known as: Bitter herb, feverwort
Latin name: *Centaurium erythraea, C. umbellatum* (synonym)
Family: Gentianaceae
Part used: Flowering tops
Usage: Centaury is a powerful alterative and cholagogue. It stimulates the appetite and cleanses the liver.
Dosage: ½ cup of tea three times daily; 15 to 40 drops of tincture three times daily
Energetics: Bitter, cold, dry
Concerns: Avoid during pregnancy. Otherwise it's safe when used appropriately. Centaury is very bitter, so it's best to take it as a tincture or capsule.

Chamomile, German

Also known as: Manzanilla, true chamomile
Latin name: *Matricaria recutita*
Family: Asteraceae
Part used: Flowers
Usage: Chamomile is a time-honored traditional medicinal herb that acts as a nerve restorative, antispasmodic, nervine, sedative, and tonic. It offers exceptional calming properties and can be used to relieve anxiety, hysteria, insomnia, pain, nightmares, restlessness, tremors, stress, and tension-related withdrawal symptoms. It cools an inflamed liver and calms headaches due to caffeine withdrawal. Chamomile helps curb the emotional need for most addictive substances and reduces cravings for alcohol and tobacco.
Dosage: 1 cup of tea three times daily; 20 to 40 drops of tincture three times daily
Energetics: Bitter, warm, moist
Concerns: Rare individuals may experience contact dermatitis from the plant.

Chaparral

Also known as: Creosote bush, greasewood
Latin name: *Larrea divaricata, L. tridentata*
Family: Zygophyllaceae
Part used: Herb
Usage: Chaparral has alterative, antioxidant, bitter, and expectorant properties. It helps remove intoxicants from the body and is especially useful for treating alcohol addictions.
Dosage: Take 2 capsules every two waking hours during withdrawal for the first five days. Then take ½ cup of tea three times daily, or 10 to 20 drops of tincture three times daily for up to five days.
Energetics: Salty, bitter, cool, dry
Concerns: Avoid during pregnancy. Avoid large doses if you're suffering from liver- or kidney-related diseases. Do not use for longer than ten days.

Cinnamon

Also known as: Cassia, sweet wood, Gui zhi
Latin name: *Cinnamomum cassia, C. zeylanicum, C. aromaticum*
Family: Lauraceae
Part used: Inner bark
Usage: Cinnamon functions as a carminative, diuretic, and thermogenic. It helps dry dampness in the body and improves circulation. It's both stimulating and calming to the nerves.
Dosage: 1 cup of tea three times daily; 30 to 50 drops of tincture three times daily
Energetics: Sweet, pungent, hot, dry
Concerns: Avoid in hot, feverish conditions. Cinnamon should be avoided by those with hemorrhoids, dry stools, or bloody urine. Avoid therapeutic dosages during pregnancy.

Cloves

Also known as: Ding xiang
Latin name: *Syzygium aromaticum*
Family: Myrtaceae
Part used: Buds
Usage: Cloves are analgesic, anesthetic, anodyne, antioxidant, expectorant, and stimulant in nature. Sucking on two whole cloves helps reduce cravings for alcohol.
Dosage: ¼ cup of tea three times daily; 10 to 20 drops of tincture three times daily
Energetics: Pungent, warm
Concerns: Safe when used appropriately.

Codonopsis

Also known as: Poor man's ginseng, bellflower, Dang shen, Tang shen
Latin name: *Codonopsis tangshen, C. pilosula*
Family: Campanulaceae
Part used: Roots
Usage: Codonopsis is an adaptogen, chi tonic, expectorant, nutritive, stimulant, and yin tonic. It helps maintain even blood sugar levels,

clears the lungs, detoxifies the blood, and tonifies the kidneys and adrenals. It can be used to treat fatigue, insomnia, memory loss, and stress.

Dosage: 1 cup of tea three times daily; 20 to 40 drops of tincture three times daily

Energetics: Sweet, warm, moist

Concerns: Safe when used appropriately.

Cola Nut

Also known as: Kola nut, bissy nut, gooroo nut

Latin name: *Cola nitida, C. acuminata*

Family: Sterculiaceae

Part used: Nuts

Usage: Cola nut has digestive, diuretic, and stimulant properties. It's used to treat alcohol, food, and drug addictions. It suppresses the appetite, aids fat metabolism, and helps relieve fatigue and mental exhaustion. A November 1974 issue of the *Journal of the American Medical Association* suggested cola nut for treating symptoms of withdrawal from alcohol, tobacco, and drug addictions.

Dosage: 1 cup of tea three times daily; 20 to 30 drops of tincture three times daily

Energetics: Bitter, cool

Concerns: Pregnant women and those with high blood pressure, heart palpitations, or peptic ulcers should avoid cola nut. Contains caffeine.

Coptis

Also known as: Goldthread, Huang lian

Latin name: *Coptis chinensis*

Family: Ranunculaceae

Part used: Rhizomes

Usage: Coptis is an antiseptic, bitter tonic, and cholagogue. It's used in traditional Chinese medicine to treat alcoholism.

Dosage: ¼ cup of tea three times daily; 5 to 10 drops of tincture three times daily

Energetics: Bitter, cold

Concerns: Avoid during pregnancy. Coptis should not be used by those suffering from gastric inflammation. It's considered at risk of becoming endangered in the wild, so don't use wildcrafted supplies.

Corydalis

Also known as: Turkey corn, Dutchman's breeches, golden smoke, Yan hu suo
Latin name: *Corydalis formosa*
Family: Papaveraceae
Part used: Rhizomes
Usage: Though only about 1 percent as strong as morphine, corydalis is as effective a pain-relieving agent, and it's not addictive. It has both analgesic and sedative properties.
Dosage: 1/4 cup of tea three times daily; 5 to 20 drops of tincture three times daily
Energetics: Acrid, bitter, warm
Concerns: Avoid during pregnancy. Use only in recommended amounts. Excessive amounts can cause tics and twitching. Therapeutic usage may cause you to test positive for opiate use in urinalysis.

Cyperus

Also known as: Sedgeroot, chufa, nut grass, Xiang fu
Latin name: *Cyperus rotundus*
Family: Cyperaceae
Part used: Rhizomes
Usage: Cyperus is analgesic, antispasmodic, sedative, and tonic. It relaxes smooth muscles and stops vomiting. It's especially helpful for treating symptoms of withdrawal from tranquilizers.
Dosage: 1 cup of tea three times daily; 20 to 40 drops of tincture three times daily
Energetics: Pungent, bitter, warm, dry
Concerns: Safe when used appropriately.

Dandelion

Also known as: Lion's tooth, blow ball, Pu gong ying
Latin name: *Taraxacum officinale*
Family: Asteraceae

Parts used: Roots, leaves

Usage: Dandelion is a cholagogue, liver tonic, and nutritive. It helps the body detoxify from drugs, tobacco, and alcohol abuse. It's a gentle liver cleanser and digestive stimulant. The root encourages metabolism of fats.

Dosage: 1 cup of tea three times daily; 30 to 60 drops of tincture three times daily

Energetics: Roots—bitter, sweet, cold; leaves—bitter, cold

Concerns: Safe when used appropriately.

Dong Quai

Also known as: Dang gui, Tang kuei

Latin name: *Angelica sinensis*

Family: Apiaceae

Part used: Roots

Usage: Dong quai has a long and honored history in traditional Chinese medicine. It functions as an alterative, antispasmodic, sedative, and yin tonic. It helps stabilize blood sugar levels, thus reducing cravings and supporting calmer moods. It also builds the blood and improves circulation. It's said to foster feelings of compassion.

Dosage: 1 cup of tea three times daily; 20 to 40 drops of tincture three times daily

Energetics: Sweet, pungent, bitter, warm, moist

Concerns: Avoid during pregnancy unless recommended by a health professional. Dong quai should not be used by those with diarrhea, poor digestion, or bloating. It may increase menstrual flow. Do not use in conjunction with blood-thinning medications.

Ephedra

Also known as: Ma huang

Latin name: *Ephedra sinica, E. distachya, E. equisetina, E. gerardiana, E. intermedia*

Family: Ephedraceae

Part used: Stems

Usage: Ephedra is a decongestant, stimulant, and thermogenic. Its active constituents include ephedrine and pseudoephedrine, which mimic the effects of epinephrine, causing vasoconstriction of the nasal mucosa, bronchial dilation, and cardiac stimulation. It helps reduce hunger and energizes the body. As a nonaddictive stimulant, ephedra can help addicts—such as those addicted to nicotine or amphetamines—let go of their addictions.

Dosage: 1 cup of tea twice daily; 20 to 30 drops of tincture three times daily

Energetics: Sweet, pungent, warm, dry

Concerns: Pregnant or nursing women and children should avoid ephedra. Ephedra should also be avoided by those suffering from anorexia, high blood pressure, debilitation, heart disease, hyperthyroid conditions, diabetes, prostatitis, hepatitis, glaucoma, insomnia, or poor digestion as well as anyone using MAO-inhibiting drugs. Large concentrated doses have been known to cause heart palpitations, insomnia, vertigo, anxiety, and even death. Excessive use can weaken the kidneys and lungs. Take early in the day to avoid sleeplessness. Long-term use can leave you feeling depleted.

Fennel

Also known as: Finocchio, Xiao hue xiang

Latin name: *Foeniculum vulgare*

Family: Apiaceae

Part used: Seeds

Usage: Fennel seeds are antispasmodic, carminative, diuretic, expectorant, laxative, and sedative; they serve as chi and stomach tonics. They can be helpful for those in the withdrawal stage. Fennel seeds are naturally sweet, which helps stabilize blood sugar levels and thereby decreases the desire for sweets, alcohol, and drugs. Fennel also improves energy.

Dosage: 1 cup of tea three times daily; 10 to 30 drops of tincture three times daily

Energetics: Pungent, sweet, warm, dry

Concerns: Fennel is safe when used appropriately, as described here. However, large doses can stimulate the nervous system.

Fenugreek

Also known as: Greek hay, Hu lu ba, Methi (Sanskrit)

Latin name: *Trigonella foenum-gracum*

Family: Fabaceae

Part used: Seeds

Usage: Fenugreek seeds have alterative, expectorant, rejuvenative, and restorative properties. They are harmonizing and demulcent in nature. Fenugreek helps remove drug residues from the body and is especially helpful for those trying to give up tobacco.

Dosage: 1 cup of tea three times daily; 20 to 60 drops of tincture three times daily

Energetics: Bitter, warm

Concerns: Avoid during pregnancy. Diabetics should consult with a health professional before using.

Feverfew

Also known as: Featherfew, febrifuge plant, wild quinine

Latin name: *Tanacetum parthenium, Chrysanthemum parthenium*

Family: Asteraceae

Parts used: Flowers, leaves

Usage: Feverfew is an antispasmodic, nervine, and tonic. It was recommended by the famous seventeenth-century herbalist Nicholas Culpepper for treatment of alcoholism.

Dosage: 1 cup of tea three times daily; 10 to 40 drops of tincture three times daily

Energetics: Bitter, warm, dry

Concerns: Individuals have reported mouth and tongue irritation from feverfew, although this is rare. Avoid during pregnancy or if you are using blood-thinning medications. Otherwise it's safe if used appropriately.

Garcinia

Also known as: Malabar tamarind, goraka

Latin name: *Garcinia cambogia, G. indica, G. atriviridis*

Family: Clusiaceae

Part used: Fruit rind

Usage: Garcinia is an antiseptic, appetite suppressant, astringent, digestive, and thermogenic. It helps curb hunger, aids in metabolism of fats, stabilizes blood sugar levels, and enhances digestion. Garcinia also appears to improve the body's ability to burn calories.

Dosage: 3 capsules three times daily

Energetics: Sour, warm

Concerns: Those allergic to citric acid (such as that found in citrus fruits and tomatoes) may have sensitivities to garcinia. Avoid during pregnancy and nursing.

Garlic

Also known as: Da suan, Rashona (Sanskrit)

Latin name: *Allium sativum*

Family: Liliaceae

Part used: Bulbs

Usage: Garlic has potent alterative, antibacterial, antioxidant, and antispasmodic properties. It's especially useful when eaten raw or taken in capsule form for clearing out the lungs.

Dosage: 1 clove eaten three times daily; 5 to 25 drops of tincture three times daily; 1 to 2 capsules three times daily

Energetics: Pungent, hot, dry

Concerns: Excessive use can cause people to become irritable and angry and can irritate the stomach and kidneys. Some people are allergic to garlic. Avoid large doses during the first three months of nursing, because it can cause the milk to be unpalatable for infants. Avoid therapeutic doses during pregnancy.

Gentian

Also known as: Bitter root, Qin jiao

Latin name: *Gentiana lutea, G. macrophylla*

Family: Gentianaceae

Part used: Roots˙

Usage: Gentian functions as an alterative, bitter tonic, and cholagogue. It dispels the desire to smoke or eat sugar and helps remove drug residues from the body.

Dosage: ¼ cup of tea three times daily; 10 to 20 drops of tincture three times daily; 1 small piece of the root eaten three times daily.

Energetics: Bitter, cold, dry

Concerns: Avoid in cases of ulcers and gastrointestinal irritation. Sensitive individuals may experience headaches. Large amounts may cause nausea and vomiting. Avoid during pregnancy. Gentian is considered at risk of becoming endangered in the wild, so don't use wildcrafted supplies.

Ginger

Also known as: Gan jiang

Latin name: *Zingiber officinale*

Family: Zingiberaceae

Part used: Roots

Usage: Ginger is an analgesic, antiemetic, antioxidant, expectorant, stimulant, and thermogenic. It improves digestion and circulation, especially to the lungs, which is helpful for clearing out residues left from smoking tobacco. It's used to treat alcohol-related gastritis and nausea from drug and alcohol withdrawal.

Dosage: ½ cup of tea four times daily; 15 drops of tincture three times daily

Energetics: Pungent, sweet, hot, dry

Concerns: Avoid large amounts in conditions of acne and eczema. Discontinue if heartburn occurs. Otherwise it's safe when used appropriately.

Ginkgo

Also known as: Maidenhair tree, Yin hsing

Latin name: *Ginkgo biloba*

Family: Ginkgoaceae

Part used: Leaves

Usage: Ginkgo is an antioxidant, cerebral tonic, kidney tonic, and rejuvenative. It improves cerebral blood flow and helps recovery of impaired memory function. It can be used to treat anxiety, dementia, and depression.

Dosage: 1 cup of tea three times daily; 20 to 40 drops of tincture three times daily

Energetics: Sweet, bitter, neutral, dry

Concerns: Side effects are rare, though headache and gastrointestinal complaints have been reported.

Ginseng, Chinese and Korean

Also known as: Ren shen

Latin name: *Panax ginseng*

Family: Araliaceae

Part used: Roots

Usage: Chinese and Korean ginseng functions as a chi tonic, rejuvenative, and restorative. It nourishes the adrenal glands and nerves, relieves stress and exhaustion, and improves physical and mental energy. It also improves debility provoked by long-term substance abuse and helps protect the body from the damaging effects of drugs and alcohol. It's especially helpful for those struggling to give up caffeine.

Dosage: 1 cup of tea three times daily; 20 to 60 drops of tincture three times daily

Energetics: Sweet, bitter, warm

Concerns: Avoid in hot conditions such as inflammation, fever, and high blood pressure. Avoid during pregnancy. Avoid prolonged use for children.

Ginseng, American

Also known as: Ren shen

Latin name: *Panax quinquefolius*

Family: Araliaceae

Part used: Roots

Usage: American ginseng offers the same benefits as Chinese ginseng. American ginseng is ideal for alcoholics to use, because it's cooler than the Chinese variety.

Energetics: Sweet, bitter, neutral

Concerns: Safe when used appropriately. American ginseng is at risk of becoming endangered in the wild, so don't use wildcrafted supplies.

Goldenseal

Also known as: Yellow pucoon, yellow root, ground raspberry
Latin name: *Hydrastis canadensis*
Family: Ranunculaceae
Part used: Roots, rhizomes
Usage: Goldenseal is an alterative, anticatarrhal, bitter, and cholagogue. It removes dampness and stagnation and cleanses drug residues from the kidneys and blood. It can be used to treat alcoholism—especially when combined with cayenne—and tobacco addiction.

Dosage: 1/2 cup of tea three times daily; 20 to 60 drops of tincture three times daily
Energetics: Bitter, cold, dry
Concerns: Use only the dried plant. Goldenseal is recommended for short-term use only, because long-term use can destroy beneficial intestinal flora and reduce B-vitamin assimilation. Avoid during pregnancy and in cases of high blood pressure. Large amounts may cause diarrhea. Goldenseal is at risk of becoming endangered, so don't use wildcrafted supplies.

Though many people have promoted goldenseal as a way to flush the urine and cause negative drug test readings, there is no validity to these claims. The myth has greatly contributed to making goldenseal an endangered species due to its difficult cultivation and overuse.

Gotu Kola

Also known as: Brahmi, Indian pennywort, Chi-hsing
Latin name: *Centella asiatica*
Family: Apiaceae
Part used: Herb
Usage: Gotu kola functions as an alterative, antispasmodic, cerebral tonic, nervine, and rejuvenative. It's of particular use as a nerve and brain restorative. It lifts the spirits from depression, clears toxins from the brain and disturbed emotions from the liver, and helps calm excessive fire in the mind. Gotu kola is used in Ayurvedic medicine to treat Kapha and Pitta types with addictions.

Dosage: ½ cup of tea three times daily; 15 to 30 drops of tincture three times daily

Energetics: Bitter, sweet, cool

Concerns: Large doses may cause headache, vertigo, itching, and loss of consciousness. In the recommended dosages gotu kola is perfectly safe to use.

Green Tea

Also known as: Cha

Latin name: *Camellia sinensis*

Family: Theaceae

Part used: Leaves

Usage: Green tea is an analgesic, antioxidant, decongestant, and stimulant. It clears the mind and calms the spirit. It also aids fat metabolism, aids digestion, curbs appetite, and energizes the body and mind. In traditional Chinese medicine green tea is said to strengthen the spleen and inhibit dampness.

Dosage: 1 cup of tea as desired

Energetics: Bitter, sweet, cool

Concerns: Green tea contains caffeine, so excessive use can cause nervous irritability. Pregnant and nursing mothers as well as those suffering from ulcers should avoid it.

Grindelia

Also known as: Gumweed, rosinweed, August flower, asthma weed

Latin name: *Grindelia robusta, G. squarrosa*

Family: Asteraceae

Part used: Herb

Usage: Grindelia has antispasmodic, expectorant, and sedative properties. It increases lung capacity, relieves coughing, and promotes cleansing of tobacco residue from the lungs.

Dosage: ¼ cup of tea three times daily; 5 to 30 drops of tincture three times daily

Energetics: Pungent, bitter, warm, moist

Concerns: Those with a history of heart problems should avoid large dosages. Large amounts can irritate the kidneys and stomach.

Gymnema

Also known as: Gurmar
Latin name: *Gymnema sylvestre*
Family: Asclepiadaceae
Parts used: Leaves, roots
Usage: Gymnema helps reduce cravings for sweets. It enhances insulin production and stabilizes blood sugar levels.
Dosage: 1 cup of tea three times daily; 2 capsules three times daily, 30 to 40 drops of tincture three times daily.
Energetics: Sweet, cool
Concerns: Diabetics should consult with a health care professional before using gymnema, because it can alter insulin requirements.

Hawthorn

Also known as: May blossom, white thorn, Shan zha
Latin name: *Crataegus oxyacantha, C. laevigata, C. monogyna, C. pinnatifida*
Family: Rosaceae
Parts used: Leaves, flowers, berries
Usage: Hawthorn is a tonic for both the emotional and the physical heart. It reduces blood fat and improves circulation, the metabolic process, and the body's ability to use oxygen.
Dosage: ½ cup of tea three times daily; 15 to 30 drops of tincture three times daily
Energetics: Flowers—cool; berries—sour, warm, dry
Concerns: If you're taking heart medications, consult with your health care practitioner before taking hawthorn, because it can potentiate the medications' effect. Use with caution in cases of colitis and ulcers. Otherwise it's safe when used appropriately.

Hops

Also known as: Ch-ku-tsao
Latin name: *Humulus lupulus*
Family: Cannabaceae
Part used: Strobiles
Usage: Hops, the sedative ingredient in beer, have anodyne, antispas-

modic, hypnotic, muscle relaxant, nervine, sedative, and soporific properties. Hops soothe nerves, quiet coughs, prevent nightmares, and calm tremors caused by drug and alcohol withdrawal. Hops can be used as a sedative for restlessness, anxiety, hysteria, stress, and insomnia. Native Americans used hops to curb desire for alcohol, and they can also be helpful for those trying to beat addictions to tranquilizers. For insomnia or nighttime restlessness, make a hops sachet and slip it into your pillowcase.

Dosage: ½ cup of tea three times daily; 15 to 30 drops of tincture three times daily

Energetics: Bitter, cold, dry

Concerns: Avoid during pregnancy and in cases of depression. The fresh plant may cause dermatitis in some individuals.

Horsetail

Also known as: Shavegrass, scouring rush, Mu zei

Latin name: *Equisetum arvense, E. telmateia, E. hyemale*

Family: Equisetaceae

Part used: Herb

Usage: Horsetail is very rich in trace minerals and functions as an alterative, diuretic, and nutritive. It can help remove drug residues from the body.

Dosage: ½ cup of tea three times daily; 15 to 30 drops of tincture three times daily

Energetics: Sweet, bitter, cool, dry

Concerns: To minimize selenium levels, use only horsetail collected in the springtime. Large amounts can cause a vitamin B1 deficiency. Those with kidney disease should avoid large dosages.

Ho Shou Wu

Also known as: Fo-ti, Chinese knotweed

Latin name: *Polygonum multiflorum*

Family: Polygonaceae

Part used: Roots

Usage: Ho shou wu is an alterative, analgesic, antispasmodic, chi tonic, rejuvenative, and yin tonic. It functions as a nerve restorative and can lift the spirits, calm anxiety, and aid sleep. It also nourishes the kidneys.

Dosage: ¼ cup of tea four times daily; 15 to 30 drops of tincture three times daily

Energetics: Bitter, sweet, warm

Concerns: Avoid during bouts of diarrhea.

Hyssop

Latin name: *Hyssopus officinalis*

Family: Lamiaceae

Part used: Herb

Usage: Hyssop has antispasmodic, diaphoretic, expectorant, and tonic properties. It calms the spirit and relieves anxiety and hysteria. It can also help remove drug residues from the body.

Dosage: ½ cup of tea three times daily; 15 to 30 drops of tincture three times daily

Energetics: Bitter, pungent, warm, dry

Concerns: Avoid during pregnancy. Hyssop should not be used by those with epilepsy or high blood pressure.

Indian Pipe

Also known as: Ghost flower, convulsion root

Latin name: *Monotropa uniflora*

Family: Ericaceae

Part used: Roots

Usage: Indian pipe is an anodyne, antispasmodic, nervine, sedative, and tonic. It's especially helpful for encouraging sound, restful sleep.

Dosage: 1 cup of tea three times daily; 20 to 30 drops of tincture three times daily. For short-term use only (up to ten days).

Energetics: Bitter, cold, dry

Concerns: Not commercially cultivated and wild products need to be collected sparingly.

Jujube Date

Also known as: Chinese date, Da zao

Latin name: *Zizyphus jujuba*

Family: Rhamnaceae

Part used: Fruit

Usage: Jujube date functions as a chi tonic, expectorant, liver tonic, nervine, nutritive, rejuvenative, and yin tonic. It supports the adrenal glands, calms the spirit, and relieves anxiety, depression, fatigue, moodiness, and stress. Jujube date can also nourishes a nervous system that has been damaged by addiction abuse.

Dosage: 1 cup of tea three times daily; 20 to 40 drops of tincture three times daily

Energetics: Sweet, warm, moist

Concerns: Avoid in damp conditions, such as bloating, and in cases of intestinal parasites. Otherwise it's safe when used appropriately.

Kava Kava

Latin name: *Piper methysticum*

Family: Piperaceae

Parts used: Roots, upper rhizomes

Usage: Kava is used as an analgesic, antispasmodic, cerebral depressant, euphoric, and sedative. It lifts depression, calms fear and anxiety, and helps relieve pain. It can be combined with valerian to aid in reducing withdrawal symptoms from tobacco and tranquilizers.

Dosage: ¼ cup of tea three times daily; 15 to 30 drops of tincture three times daily

Energetics: Pungent, bitter, hot

Concerns: Excessive use can dilate the pupils and impair walking and driving. Even small doses can cause your mouth and tongue to feel numb temporarily and cause other body parts to feel rubbery. Avoid during pregnancy and nursing. Kava is at risk of becoming endangered in the wild, so don't use wildcrafted supplies.

Kudzu

Also known as: Kuzu, Ge gen

Latin name: *Pueraria lobata, P. thomsonii*

Family: Fabaceae

Parts used: Roots, flowers

Usage: Kudzu functions as an antispasmodic, demulcent, diaphoretic, restorative, and tonic. It decreases alcohol cravings, increases energy, and helps balance the hormonal system. Kudzu is an ancient Chinese remedy for drunkenness. It causes acetaldehyde to build up faster in the blood so that drinking becomes less pleasant, and lesser amounts of alcohol cause greater hangovers. In one study hamsters offered a choice of water or alcohol chose alcohol. After having been given kudzu, however, they chose water.

Dosage: 1 cup of tea three times daily; 2 capsules three times daily
Energetics: Sweet, bitter, pungent, cool, moist
Concerns: Safe when used appropriately.

Lavender

Latin name: *Lavendula officinalis, L. angustifolia, L. latifolia, L. stoechas*
Family: Lamiaceae
Part used: Flowers
Usage: Aromatic lavender has analgesic, antidepressant, antispasmodic, cholagogue, nervine, and sedative properties. It's well known for calming the spirit, but it also curbs the desire for alcohol, caffeine, and tobacco and is especially helpful for withdrawal from alcohol or sedatives.
Dosage: ½ cup of tea three times daily; 30 to 40 drops of tincture three times daily
Energetics: Bitter, cool, dry
Concerns: Safe when used appropriately.

Lemon Balm

Also known as: Bee balm
Latin name: *Melissa officinalis*
Family: Lamiaceae
Part used: Herb
Usage: Lemon balm is a gentle, uplifting healer with antispasmodic, hypotensive, nervine, rejuvenative, sedative, and tonic properties. It's especially helpful during the withdrawal and detoxification period.
Dosage: 1 cup of tea three times daily; 20 to 40 drops of tincture three times daily
Energetics: Sour, pungent, cold, dry
Concerns: Safe when used as directed.

Licorice

Also known as: Gan cao, Yashti mudhu (Sanskrit)

Latin name: *Glycyrrhiza glabra, G. echinata, G. uralensis*

Family: Fabaceae

Part used: Roots

Usage: Licorice is an adrenal and chi tonic, antispasmodic, antitussive, demulcent, expectorant, nutritive, and rejuvenative. It can be used to treat fatigue, stress, and coughs and helps induce a feeling of peace, calm, and harmony. Licorice is especially helpful for those struggling to give up addictions to drugs, alcohol, tobacco, sugar, and caffeine. It keeps blood sugar levels even and can be of great help during the withdrawal and detoxification period.

Dosage: ½ cup of tea three times daily; 30 to 60 drops of tincture three times daily

Energetics: Sweet, bitter, neutral, moist

Concerns: Those with diabetes, rapid heartbeat, hypertension, or severe edema as well as those taking digoxin drugs should avoid licorice. It should also be avoided during pregnancy. Excessive use can cause sodium retention and potassium depletion.

Linden

Also known as: Lime tree, basswood

Latin name: *Tilia platyphylla, T. americana, T. cordata, T. eurpoaea*

Family: Tiliaceae

Parts used: Leaves, flowers

Usage: Linden has antispasmodic, choleretic, expectorant, hypotensive, nervine, sedative, and tonic properties. It's known for its ability to calm the spirit and relieve stress and anxiety.

Dosage: 1 cup of tea three times daily; 20 to 40 drops of tincture three times daily

Energetics: Pungent, sweet, warm, dry

Concerns: Large doses of *T. americana* have been reported to cause nausea in some individuals. Linden is safe when used appropriately.

Lobelia

Also known as: Emetic weed, Indian tobacco, pukeweed
Latin name: *Lobelia inflata, L. siphilitica, L. cardinalis, L. chinensis*
Family: Campanulaceae
Parts used: Leaves, flowers, seeds
Usage: Lobelia is an antispasmodic, a nervine, and a respiratory stimulant. It's often used to treat bronchial spasms, coughs, and muscle spasms. In small doses lobelia is relaxing, and in large doses it can be stimulating. It's used for alcohol, tobacco, and tranquilizer addictions. One of its constituents, lobeline, has a nicotine-like effect and can thus ease withdrawal symptoms for smokers.
Dosage: ¼ cup of tea three times daily; 10 to 15 drops of tincture three times daily. When a nicotine craving strikes, take 5 drops (*not* dropperfuls) of tincture under the tongue.
Energetics: Bitter, pungent, warm
Concerns: Use only in small doses—about one-fifth the dose for other herbs. Large doses can cause vomiting. Lobelia should be avoided by those with high blood pressure and those prone to fainting. Lobelia is considered at risk of becoming endangered in the wild, so don't use wildcrafted supplies.

Magnolia

Also known as: Hou po
Latin name: *Magnolia officinalis*
Family: Magnoliaceae
Part used: Bark
Usage: Magnolia bark functions as an analgesic, antispasmodic, aromatic, bronchial dilator, decongestant, expectorant, and stimulant. It can help you break the tobacco habit. In traditional Chinese medicine it's said to move stagnant chi and dry dampness.
Dosage: ½ cup of tea three times daily; 30 to 50 drops of tincture three times daily
Energetics: Bitter, pungent, warm, dry
Concerns: Large amounts can cause vertigo.

Marjoram

Latin name: *Majorana hortensis, Origanum majorana*
Family: Lamiaceae
Part used: Herb
Usage: Marjoram has anti-inflammatory, antioxidant, antispasmodic, aromatic, cholagogue, diaphoretic, expectorant, and stimulant properties. It's excellent for smokers trying to kick the tobacco habit: just drink ½ cup of marjoram tea every time you desire a cigarette. Marjoram will dry the throat and diminish the pleasure derived from smoking.
Dosage: 1 cup of tea three times daily; 10 to 30 drops of tincture three times daily
Energetics: Pungent, warm
Concerns: Avoid therapeutic dosages during pregnancy.

Marsh Mallow

Latin name: *Althaea officinalis*
Family: Malvaceae
Parts used: Roots, leaves, flowers
Usage: Marsh mallow is an alterative, demulcent, expectorant, nutritive, rejuvenative, and yin tonic. It's used to treat coughs, and in traditional Chinese medicine it's said to moisten the lungs and the kidneys.
Dosage: 1 cup of tea three times daily; 20 to 40 drops of tincture three times daily
Energetics: Sweet, cool, moist
Concerns: Safe when used appropriately.

Milk Thistle

Latin name: *Silybum marianum*
Family: Asteraceae
Part used: Seeds
Usage: Milk thistle seed has antidepressant, antioxidant, bitter tonic, cholagogue, demulcent, and hepato-protective properties. It stimulates protein synthesis in the liver and improves breakdown of

waste products. It's used to treat cirrhosis of the liver and liver damage caused by drugs and alcohol.

Dosage: 15 to 25 drops of tincture three times daily

Energetics: Sweet, bitter, cool

Concerns: Safe when used appropriately.

Motherwort

Also known as: Lion's ear, Tsan-tsai

Latin name: *Leonurus cardiaca*

Family: Lamiaceae

Part used: Herb

Usage: Motherwort is known to be an antispasmodic, cardiotonic, circulatory stimulant, diuretic, hypotensive, nervine, rejuvenative, sedative, and vasodilator. It calms heart palpitations caused by anxiety and helps relieve exhaustion, depression, and hysteria.

Dosage: ½ cup of tea three times daily; 10 to 20 drops of tincture three times daily

Energetics: Pungent, bitter, cool, dry

Concerns: Avoid in cases of excessive menstrual bleeding. Motherwort should not be used during pregnancy. The fresh plant may cause contact dermatitis in some people.

Mugwort

Latin name: *Artemesia vulgaris, A. douglasiana, A. lactiflora*

Family: Asteraceae

Part used: Herb

Usage: Mugwort is an antispasmodic, bitter tonic, cholagogue, and nervine. It's traditionally used to treat anorexia, depression, and hysteria, and it's especially useful in helping the body detoxify from tranquilizers.

Dosage: ¼ cup of tea three times daily; 10 to 20 drops of tincture three times daily

Energetics: Bitter, pungent, cool, dry

Concerns: Use only in the dosages recommended here; larger amounts can adversely affect the nervous system. Don't use for long periods of time (more than ten days). Avoid during pregnancy.

Mullein

Also known as: Velvet dock, witch's candle
Latin name: *Verbascum thapsus, V. densiflorum, V. phlomoides*
Family: Scrophulariaceae
Parts used: Leaves, flowers
Usage: Mullein functions as an antispasmodic, demulcent, expectorant, nervine, sedative, and yin tonic. It cleans the lungs and lymph vessels and helps remove drug residues from the body. It's traditionally used to overcome tobacco addictions.
Dosage: 1 cup of tea three times daily; 30 to 60 drops of tincture three times daily
Energetics: Sweet, bitter, cool, moist
Concerns: Safe when used appropriately.

Nettle

Also known as: Stinging nettle
Latin name: *Urtica dioica, U. californica, U. urens, U. gracilis, U. holosericea*
Family: Urticaceae
Part used: Leaves
Usage: Nettle is an adrenal tonic, alterative, cholagogue, circulatory stimulant, diuretic, expectorant, kidney tonic, nutritive, respiratory tonic, and thyroid tonic. It's rich in minerals and makes a nourishing tonic for convalescence. It helps relieve allergies and improves metabolism. Nettle is also a folk remedy for reducing cellulite and aiding weight loss.
Dosage: 1 cup of tea three times daily; 20 to 40 drops of tincture three times daily
Energetics: Bitter, salty, cool
Concerns: Avoid eating the raw plant. When adding nettle to your food, choose young, tender leaves; the older leaves can be irritating to the kidneys. Otherwise it's safe when used appropriately.

Oat Seed, Oatstraw

Also known as: Yen-mai
Latin name: *Avena sativa, A. fatua*

Family: Poaceae

Part used: Spikelets (best), herb

Usage: Oat seed is the whole seed with the milky juice inside and most herbalists prefer it. Oatstraw is next best and more commonly available. *Avena* has antidepressant, antispasmodic, cerebral tonic, nervine, nutritive, and rejuvenative properties. It calms and strengthens the nerves, lessens anxiety, and decreases the desire for alcohol, caffeine, and tobacco. In a study conducted at Ruchill Hospital in Glasgow, Scotland, a tincture of oatstraw was given in oral doses of 5 milliliters to a group of heavy smokers. A second group was given a placebo. The first group had been smoking an average of 19.5 cigarettes daily before entering the study; after a month of taking oatstraw tincture, that number had decreased to 5.7 cigarettes daily. The placebo group had been smoking 16.5 cigarettes at the beginning of the study; after a month, usage had actually increased to 16.7 cigarettes daily.

Dosage: 1 cup of tea three times daily; 20 to 40 drops of tincture three times daily

Energetics: Sweet, cool, moist

Concerns: Safe when used appropriately.

Ophiopogon

Also known as: Japanese lily turf, Mai men Dong

Latin name: *Ophiopogon japonicus*

Family: Liliaceae

Part used: Roots

Usage: Ophiopogon is a demulcent, expectorant, nutritive, restorative, sedative, and yin tonic. It calms irritability and relieves constipation and mouth dryness.

Dosage: 1 cup of tea three times daily; 30 to 60 drops of tincture three times daily

Energetics: Sweet, bitter, cool, moist

Concerns: Avoid in cases of diarrhea and nasal congestion.

Orange Peel

Also known as: Chen pi

Latin name: *Citrus reticulata*

Family: Rutaceae

Usage: Orange peel has aromatic, bitter, cholagogue, expectorant, sedative, and tonic properties. In traditional Chinese medicine it's said to help move liver stagnation and clear lung congestion.

Dosage: 1 cup of tea three times daily; 20 to 40 drops of tincture three times daily

Energetics: Pungent, bitter, warm, sour, cool, dry

Concerns: Avoid during pregnancy except under the recommendation of a health professional.

Osha

Also known as: Empress of the dark forest, porter's lovage, bear medicine, mountain carrot

Latin name: *Ligusticum poterii, L. apifolium, L. californicum*

Family: Apiaceae

Part used: Roots

Usage: Osha is an anesthetic, aromatic, circulatory stimulant, diaphoretic, expectorant, and hypotensive. It helps remove tobacco pollutants from lungs, relieves coughing, and soothes irritated lung tissue. It's often burned as incense for purification rituals.

Dosage: ½ cup of tea three times daily; 10 to 30 drops of tincture three times daily

Energetics: Pungent, warm, bitter, dry

Concerns: Avoid during pregnancy. Osha is at risk of becoming endangered in the wild, so don't use wildcrafted supplies.

Parsley

Latin name: *Petroselinum crispum*

Family: Apiaceae

Parts used: Leaves, roots

Usage: Parsley has alterative, antioxidant, antispasmodic, carminative, diuretic, expectorant, nutritive, and sedative properties. It helps cleanse the kidneys and the leaves are high in chlorophyll, making it an excellent agent for detoxification and recommended for use during withdrawal. Parsley is a traditional remedy for alcoholism.

Dosage: 1 cup of tea three times daily; 30 to 60 drops of tincture three times daily

Energetics: Sweet, neutral

Concerns: Avoid therapeutic dosages (anything more than what you use to season your food) during pregnancy and in cases of kidney inflammation.

Passionflower

Also known as: Maypop, flower of the five wounds
Latin name: *Passiflora incarnata*
Family: Passifloraceae
Part used: Herb
Usage: Passionflower functions as an antispasmodic, hypnotic, hypotensive, nervine, and sedative. It quiets the nervous system, calms the spirit, and relieves restlessness, stress, insomnia, anger, anxiety, convulsions, and hysteria. It's often recommended for treating alcohol, tobacco, and tranquilizer addictions. Its potent calming properties can be useful for someone in the withdrawal period.
Dosage: ½ cup of tea three times daily; 15 to 60 drops of tincture three times daily
Energetics: Bitter, cool
Concerns: Large doses can cause nausea and vomiting. Avoid large doses during pregnancy. Otherwise it's safe when used appropriately.

Peppermint

Latin name: *Mentha piperita*
Family: Lamiaceae
Part used: Herb
Usage: Peppermint is an analgesic, anodyne, antidepressant, antispasmodic, aromatic, cholagogue, diaphoretic, nerve restorative, stimulant, tonic, and vasodilator. It functions as a mild stimulant, both opening and relaxing for the mind, and it helps clean out the lungs. Peppermint can be used to treat coughs, headache, and nausea. It's often recommended to treat drug and nicotine addictions and to soothe and uplift the spirit of those in the withdrawal period.
Dosage: 1 cup of tea three times daily; 10 to 50 drops of tincture three times daily
Energetics: Pungent, cool, dry
Concerns: Safe when used appropriately.

Plantain

Also known as: White man's footsteps, waybread, broad leaf plantain, ribwort

Latin name: *Plantago major, P. lanceolata, P. media*

Family: Plataginaceae

Part used: Leaves

Usage: Plantain is an alterative, anti-inflammatory, antispasmodic, expectorant, decongestant, demulcent, and diuretic. It clears phlegm and heat from the body and soothes irritated and inflamed tissues. In folk medicine chewing on a plantain stem is said to be a quick remedy for staving off a cigarette craving.

Dosage: 1 cup of tea three times daily; 20 to 60 drops of tincture three times daily

Energetics: Sweet, bitter, salty, cool, dry

Concerns: Safe when used appropriately.

Poria

Also known as: Indian bread, tuckahoe, hoelen, Fu ling

Latin name: *Poria cocus, Wolfiporia cocu*s

Family: Polyporaceae

Usage: Poria is a chi tonic, diuretic, expectorant, restorative, sedative, and tonic. It calms the mind and drains dampness. It's recommended for treating anxiety and insomnia and as a tonic during convalescence.

Dosage: 1 cup of tea three times daily; 40 drops of tincture three times daily

Energetics: Sweet, neutral, dry

Concerns: Safe when used appropriately.

Red Clover

Also known as: Sweet clover, trefoil, Vana-methika (Sanskrit)

Latin name: *Trifolium pratense*

Family: Fabaceae

Parts used: Young leaves, flowers

Usage: Red clover is an alterative, anti-inflammatory, antispasmodic, expectorant, and nutritive. It aids in the body's natural detoxification process and is helpful during withdrawal.

Dosage: 1 cup of tea three times daily; 20 to 40 drops of tincture three times daily

Energetics: Sweet, salty, cool

Concerns: Avoid during pregnancy.

Reishi

Also known as: Lucky fungus, Ling zhi

Latin name: *Ganoderma lucidum*

Family: Polyporaceae

Part used: Fruiting body

Usage: Reishi mushrooms are often used by Taoist monks to calm the mind and spirit. They have adaptogenic, cardiotonic, and rejuvenative properties. They are recommended to relieve anxiety, calm the nerves, and treat insomnia.

Dosage: 1 cup of tea three times daily; 20 to 40 drops of tincture three times daily

Energetics: Bland, sweet, bitter, neutral

Concerns: Safe when used appropriately. There have been rare reports of dry mouth, digestive distress, nosebleeds, and bloody stools when reishi has been used for extended periods of time (at least three to six months).

Rosemary

Latin name: *Rosmarinus officinalis*

Family: Lamiaceae

Part used: Herb

Usage: Rosemary is an antioxidant, decongestant, nervine, and rejuvenative. It helps calm anxiety, improve mental alertness, lift depression, and improve liver and lung function.

Dosage: 1 cup of tea three times daily; 15 to 30 drops of tincture three times daily

Energetics: Pungent, bitter, warm, dry

Concerns: Do not exceed the recommended dosage. Avoid therapeutic dosages (anything more than what you use to season your food) during pregnancy.

Sage

Also known as: Dalmatian sage, Shu-wei-tsao
Latin name: *Salvia officinalis*
Family: Lamiaceae
Part used: Herb
Usage: Sage functions as an antidepressant, antispasmodic, aromatic, cerebral tonic, choleretic, expectorant, nervine, nerve restorative, and rejuvenative. It helps remove drug residues from the body.
Dosage: ½ cup of tea three times daily; 15 to 30 drops of tincture three times daily
Energetics: Pungent, warm, dry
Concerns: Pregnant and nursing mothers as well as epileptics should avoid therapeutic dosages (anything more than what you use to season your food). Don't use for more than ten days.

St. John's wort

Also known as: Saint-Joan's-wort, Klamath weed, goat weed, Qian ceng lou
Latin name: *Hypericum perforatum*
Family: Hyperiaceae
Part used: Herb
Usage: St. John's wort has alterative, antidepressant, antispasmodic, cholagogue, expectorant, nerve restorative, and sedative properties. It's often used to treat depression and anxiety—both mental states that can contribute to addictions. It can be used to treat alcohol, caffeine, tobacco, and tranquilizer addictions.
Dosage: ½ cup of tea three times daily; 10 to 15 drops of tincture three times daily
Energetics: Bitter, sweet, cold, dry
Concerns: St. John's wort can cause photosensitivity in some individuals, especially those who are fair skinned. The fresh plant can

cause contact dermatitis in rare cases. St. John's wort should not be used in combination with MAO-inhibiting drugs, because it can potentiate their effects.

Sassafras

Also known as: Cinnamon wood, fennel wood, ague tree
Latin name: *Sassafras albidum*
Family: Lauraceae
Parts used: Leaves, root bark
Usage: Sassafras is an alterative, anodyne, aromatic, diaphoretic, and diuretic. Chewing its inner bark can help decrease the desire to smoke.
Dosage: ¼ cup of tea four times daily; 15 to 30 drops of tincture three times daily
Energetics: Pungent, warm
Concerns: Avoid during pregnancy and nursing. Sassafras is meant for occasional use, not as a long-term treatment. Do not exceed the recommended dosages.

Saw Palmetto

Also known as: Sabal
Latin name: *Serenoa serrulata, S. repens*
Family: Arecaceae
Part used: Berries
Usage: Saw palmetto berries have expectorant, nerve restorative, nutritive, rejuvenative, and tonic properties. They're recommended to treat alcoholism and are especially helpful in cases where a person is "wasting away."
Dosage: ½ cup of tea three times daily; 10 to 60 drops of tincture three times daily
Energetics: Pungent, sweet, warm
Concerns: There have been rare reports of saw palmetto causing stomach distress. Otherwise it's safe when used appropriately.

Schizandra

Also known as: Fruit of the five flavors, magnolia vine, Wu wei zi
Latin name: *Schisandra chinensis*
Family: Schisandraceae
Part used: Fruit
Usage: Schizandra functions as an adaptogen, antidepressant, cerebral tonic, kidney tonic, liver tonic, nerve restorative, rejuvenative, and sedative. In traditional Chinese medicine it's used to enhance physical and mental balance—to "calm the heart and quiet the spirit." Schizandra improves endurance, coordination, and concentration and helps the body better utilize oxygen. It calms anxiety and relieves depression, fatigue, irritability, and memory loss. It's often recommended as a treatment for alcoholism.
Dosage: ½ cup of tea three times daily; 20 to 30 drops of tincture three times daily
Energetics: Sour, sweet, salty, pungent, bitter, warm
Concerns: Avoid in conditions of excess heat, such as fever and infection. Schizandra may be contraindicated for those with epilepsy, intracranial pressure, or high stomach acid.

Siberian Ginseng

Also known as: Eleuthero, Ci wu jia
Latin name: *Eleutherococcus senticosus*
Family: Araliaceae
Parts used: Roots, root bark
Usage: Siberian ginseng is an adaptogen, antidepressant, antispasmodic, cardiotonic, chi tonic, and nerve restorative. It nourishes the adrenal glands, which can become exhausted from substance abuse, and helps protect the body from the toxic effects of drugs and alcohol. It can be used to treat depression, fatigue, insomnia, memory loss, nervous breakdown, and stress.
Dosage: 1 cup of tea three times daily; 20 to 40 drops of tincture three times daily
Energetics: Sweet, bitter, neutral
Concerns: Safe when used appropriately.

Skullcap

Also known as: Blue pimpernel, Quaker's hat, mad dog weed
Latin name: *Scutellaria lateriflora*
Family: Lamiaceae
Part used: Herb
Usage: Skullcap functions as an alterative, anodyne, antispasmodic, bitter tonic, cerebral tonic, nerve restorative, nervine, sedative, and yin tonic. It calms the emotions, enhances awareness, and quiets overexcitability. It can be used to treat anxiety, convulsions, delirium tremens, nightmares, pain, panic, restlessness, and withdrawal. Skullcap helps curb the emotional need and cravings for addictive substances; it's recommended for the withdrawal period of alcohol, caffeine, tobacco, and tranquilizer addictions.
Dosage: 1 cup of tea three times daily; 20 to 40 drops of tincture three times daily
Energetics: Bitter, cold, dry
Concerns: Avoid large doses during pregnancy. Otherwise it's safe when used appropriately.

Slippery Elm

Also known as: Indian elm, red elm
Latin name: *Ulmus fulva, U. rubra*
Family: Ulmaceae
Part used: Inner bark
Usage: Slippery elm bark is a demulcent, expectorant, nutritive, restorative, and yin tonic. It's calming for the spirit and gives nutritional support during convalescence. It can be made up into an easily digested gruel for those who can't hold down any food. Slippery elm also soothes irritated mucous membranes. It can help decrease tobacco cravings.
Dosage: ½ cup of tea four times daily: stir 1 teaspoon into ¼ cup of warm water and eat as a gruel
Energetics: Sweet, neutral, moist
Concerns: Safe when used appropriately. Slippery elm is at risk of becoming endangered in the wild, so don't use wildcrafted supplies.

Thyme

Also known as: Garden thyme

Latin name: *Thymus vulgaris*

Family: Lamiaceae

Part used: Herb

Usage: Thyme has antidepressant, antispasmodic, aromatic, diaphoretic, diuretic, expectorant, and rejuvenative properties. It helps cleanse the liver and lungs. Thyme is used in Russian folk medicine to treat alcoholism, and it's excellent for those struggling to give up the tobacco habit.

Dosage: ½ cup of tea three times daily; 10 to 20 drops of tincture three times daily

Energetics: Pungent, bitter, warm, dry

Concerns: Avoid therapeutic dosages (anything more than what you use to season your food) during pregnancy. Otherwise it's safe when used appropriately.

Turmeric

Also known as: Jiang huang, Haridra (Sanskrit)

Latin name: *Curcuma longa, C. aromatica, C. domestica*

Family: Zingiberaceae

Part used: Rhizomes

Usage: Turmeric is an alterative, analgesic, antioxidant, aromatic, cholagogue, circulatory stimulant, hepato-tonic, and stimulant. It helps clear negative emotions from the liver and protects the liver from the harmful effects of drug, smoke, and chemical exposure. It increases energy, improves digestion, and inhibits yeast over-growth. It's often recommended for treatment of alcoholism.

Dosage: 1 teaspoon of powder in a cup of hot water three times daily; 20 to 40 drops of tincture three times daily

Energetics: Pungent, bitter, warm

Concerns: Turmeric may cause photosensitivity in some people. Pregnant woman and those suffering from gallstones should avoid therapeutic dosages (anything more than what you use to season your food).

Uva Ursi

Also known as: Kinnikinnik, mountain cranberry, bearberry, arbutus
Latin name: *Arctostaphylos uva-ursi*
Family: Ericaceae
Part used: Leaves
Usage: Uva ursi is recommended in Russian folk medicine as a treatment for alcoholism. It's a demulcent and genitourinary antiseptic.
Dosage: 1 cup of tea three times daily; 20 to 40 drops of tincture three times daily for no more than ten days
Energetics: Bitter, pungent, cold
Concerns: Avoid during pregnancy. Uva ursi may give urine a greenish, though harmless, color. Long-term use can be constipating. If you wish to use uva ursi for more than ten days at a time, first consult with a health professional.

Valerian

Also known as: Garden heliotrope, Phu, Tagara (Sanskrit)
Latin name: *Valeriana officinalis, V. edulis, V. sitchensis, V. wallichii*
Family: Valerianaceae
Parts used: Rhizomes, roots
Usage: Valerian functions as an antispasmodic, hypnotic, muscle relaxant, nerve restorative, nervine, and sedative. It can be used as a nonaddictive substitute for those struggling to give up an addiction to sedatives, and it's also useful for treating nicotine and alcohol addictions. Valerian is very helpful during the withdrawal period, because it calms cravings and relieves anxiety, restlessness, hysteria, insomnia, and stress.
Dosage: 1 cup of tea as needed, up to three times daily; 20 to 40 drops of tincture as needed
Energetics: Pungent, bitter, warm, dry
Concerns: Pregnant women and those suffering from severe depression, low blood pressure, or hypoglycemia should avoid valerian. Large doses can cause individuals to feel lethargic. Otherwise it's safe when used appropriately.

Wild Lettuce

Also known as: Prickly lettuce, poor man's opium, lettuce opium
Latin name: *Lactuca virosa, L. serriola, L. quercina*
Family: Asteraceae
Part used: Herb
Usage: Wild lettuce has analgesic, anodyne, antitussive, expectorant, hypnotic, and sedative properties. It aids sleep, calms anxiety and restlessness, and relieves pain.
Dosage: 1 cup of tea three times daily; 20 to 40 drops of tincture three times daily
Energetics: Bitter, cool
Concerns: Avoid in cases of prostate enlargement and glaucoma. Be sure to keep the plant's fresh latex, a potential irritant, away from your eyes. Otherwise it's safe when used appropriately.

Wood Betony

Also known as: Bishop's wort
Latin name: *Stachys officinalis*
Family: Lamiaceae
Part used: Herb
Usage: Wood betony is a wonderful alterative, analgesic, antispasmodic, aromatic, bitter, cerebral tonic, circulatory stimulant, hepatotonic, nervine, and sedative. As a nerve restorative it calms the spirit, eases anxiety, and relieves exhaustion.
Dosage: 1 cup of tea twice daily; 20 to 30 drops of tincture three times daily
Energetics: Bitter, cool, dry
Concerns: Avoid large doses during pregnancy, except when recommended by a health professional for labor. Large doses can be emetic. Otherwise it's safe when used appropriately.

Yellow Dock

Also known as: Curly dock, sour dock, Chin-chiao-mai
Latin name: *Rumex crispus, R. obtusifolius*
Family: Polygonaceae

Part used: Roots

Usage: Yellow dock is an alterative, blood tonic, and cholagogue. It improves the functioning of the kidneys, liver, and lymphatic system, thus aiding the body's natural cleansing process. Use during withdrawal.

Dosage: 1/2 cup of tea four times daily; 5 to 30 drops of tincture three times daily

Energetics: Bitter, cool, dry

Concerns: Those with kidney stones should use yellow dock only in moderation.

Yerba Maté

Also known as: Maté, Paraguay tea

Latin name: *Ilex paraguariensis*

Family: Aquifoliaceae

Part used: Roasted leaves

Usage: Yerba maté is an alterative, antidepressant, antioxidant, diuretic, nerve stimulant, nutritive, rejuvenative, stimulant, and tonic. It's a healthier alternative to coffee, black tea, and amphetamines. It helps relieve fatigue and depression, brightens your general outlook on life, and can be used to curb food addictions and aid weight loss.

Dosage: 1 cup of tea as desired up to four times daily

Energetics: Warm, drying

Concerns: Do not consume yerba maté with meals, because its high tannin content can impair nutrient assimilation. Yerba maté contains mateine, which is in most circles considered identical to caffeine—although it's less likely to impair sleep or cause addiction.

Yerba Santa

Also known as: Holy herb, tar weed, consumptive weed

Latin name: *Eriodictyon californicum, E. tomentosum*

Family: Hydrophyllaceae

Parts used: Leaves, resin

Usage: Yerba santa functions as an alterative, antispasmodic, aromatic, bronchial dilator, decongestant, expectorant, and stimulant.

The gummy resin from the plant can be chewed or smoked as a tobacco substitute. It has a sweet flavor when smoked. It decreases phlegm and reduces inflammation in the lungs.

Dosage: 1 cup of tea three times daily; 20 to 40 drops of tincture three times daily

Energetics: Pungent, warm

Concerns: Safe when used appropriately. Yerba santa is considered at risk of becoming endangered in the wild, so don't use wildcrafted supplies.

Homeopathy for Addiction

Homeopathy, developed in the eighteenth century by the German physician Samuel Hahnemann, is a form of natural medicine that uses minute amounts of natural substances to cause the body to heal itself. Homeopathy has a long history of success and is practiced throughout the world. For addictions, homeopathy offers help in healing both the psychological and the physical dependencies.

To treat addictions, use homeopathic remedies in 200c (or 200x) potencies every week until the craving is gone. For the greatest effectiveness, consult with a homeopath to find the specific constitutional remedy that's right for you.

- *Absinthium* is for the patient who feels disoriented, dizzy, and depressed, possibly with hallucinations.
- *Aconitum napellus* is for the restless person who tosses about during withdrawal, feels he or she may die, or suffers from anxiety. It's especially helpful for those with alcohol and tobacco dependencies.
- *Anacardium* is for irritable people with a tendency to use violence and obscene language.
- *Apomorphia* is for the patient with nausea and low vitality who sweats and salivates a lot.
- *Arnica* is for a patient in withdrawal who feels bruised and doesn't want to be touched, and who craves solitude.

- *Arsenicum album* is for those addicted to alcohol and painkillers. These patients may tend to be hypochondriacs, to have a restless and anxious nature, and to fear being left alone. They may be prone to vomiting or diarrhea.
- *Aurum metallicum* is for the patient who has turned to an addiction due to pain from having fallen from a high level of importance. He or she may fear failure and may have a tendency to hide anger behind an arrogant attitude.
- *Avena sativa* is for nervous exhaustion and insomnia, especially as related to alcoholism.
- *Berberis* is for alcoholism.
- *Caladium seguinum* is for nicotine addictions.
- *Calcarea carbonica* is for those who are overweight and suffer from food cravings.
- *Cannabis sativa* is for the patient with a perspiring, flushed face who is overexcited and talkative, especially as related to alcoholism.
- *Capsicum frutescens* is for upset stomach, intense craving, and delirium, especially as related to alcohol withdrawal.
- *Chelidonium majus* is for jaundice and pain originating in the liver from drug abuse.
- *Coffea cruda* is for caffeine withdrawal.
- *Hyoscyamus niger* is for tremors and hysteria that alternates between laughing and crying. The patient may be paranoid, may curse and mutter, and may be resentful of those pushing him or her toward rehabilitation. *Hyoscyamus niger* is especially useful in the treatment of alcoholism and drug abuse.
- *Ignatia* is for the treatment of acute grief, shock anger, mood swings, and hysteria. The patient may suppress emotions, show changeable symptoms, and suffer from chills, thirst, and sensitivity to pain.
- *Lachesis* is for alcoholic cravings. It's especially helpful for talkative, dramatic, and emotionally intense people. They may fear they are being persecuted for their drug addiction; anger and rage are at the roots of their addiction. They often have a biting tongue.
- *Lycopodium* is for the young, successful employee who feels trapped in a "safe" job yet longs to live on the wild side and now turns to drugs or alcohol.

- *Nux vomica* is for the addictions of a Type-A personality, and for the workaholic with underlying tensions that contribute to addictions; he or she may be angry, jealous, impatient, and overly sensitive. *Nux vomica* helps reduce underlying tensions and relax the nervous system. It relieves headache, irritability, frightening visions, and tremors.

> *Nux vomica* is considered *the* addiction remedy. It can help users learn to say no to addictive substances, and it's therapeutic during the withdrawal period as well.

- *Petroleum* is for the low-energy alcoholic who can never refuse a drink and talks a lot when drunk.
- *Quercus* is for alcoholism and alcohol craving.
- *Staphysagria* is for the addict who suppresses anger but is on the verge of erupting. It's especially helpful for victims of physical and sexual abuse. Patients may experience nausea and uneasiness. It's also helpful for treating nicotine addictions.
- *Stramonium* is for withdrawal so severe that it causes convulsions, hallucinations, incessant talking, swearing, and lewd behavior. It's especially helpful for treating alcoholism.
- *Sulphuricum acidum* is for chronic alcoholics who think they are superior to everyone else and who are untidy and philosophical. They may have a red nose.
- *Syphilinum* is for inherited alcoholic tendencies.
- *Tabacum* is for tobacco cravings.
- *Veratrum album* is for the workaholic with digestive problems and a persistent feeling of being thirsty.
- *Zincum metallicum* is for withdrawal in late stages where twitching, depression, irritability, and restlessness occur.

Massage Therapy and Bodywork

Massage and other forms of bodywork can relax the body and mind, improve circulation, and energize your life. These therapies are tremendously helpful for those struggling to give up addictions. For mental health and physical well-being, I recommend getting full-body massages whenever possible!

Patent Medicines for Addictions

There are two Chinese patent medicines that I recommend for treating addictions. Free and Easy Wanderer (Xiao Yao Wan), also known as Bupleurum Sedative Pills, helps detoxify the body while promoting relaxation, stabilizing blood sugar, and functioning as a chi tonic. Dong Quai and Peony Combination is a good formula to use in overcoming alcoholism. It improves fatigue, depression, and liver health; builds the blood; and helps the body adapt to stressful situations.

If you don't have time for a full-body massage, consider a head massage. The head is a sensitive and nerve-rich area, so head massages are beneficial for everyone, and particularly for those with addictions. Here's how to give one: The patient should lie flat on his or her back. Sit behind the patient, taking the weight of the skull in your hands. Making small circular motions with the pads of your fingers, work around the base of the skull and up into the hair. Move on up to the temple regions, then lightly over the sinus regions, down the sides of the nose, and over the mouth. Combine smooth strokes and light taps on head and face.

Foot massage is also helpful: it can bring energy down from the head, keep you grounded, and help you feel warm.

Cranial sacral work, biofeedback, hypnosis, Alexander Work, and chiropractic are other healing therapies that can soothe your spirit and help your body heal.

Acupuncture and Acupressure

Acupuncture stimulates detoxification, promotes a heightened sense of relaxation, and encourage endorphin production, which makes it an excellent tool for overcoming addiction. Many health insurance companies will pay for visits to an acupuncturist; check with your provider for more information.

Acupressure is a form of acupuncture that can be practiced at home as well as by a professional. It's like a potent form of massage: the acupressurist presses acupuncture points, stimulating the body's healing abilities without using needles.

To deter substance cravings, press the following acupressure points firmly with your thumb or fingertip:

- SI19, at the ear opening in the hollow formed by the mouth being open
- LI4, at the back of the hand where the thumb and index finger meet

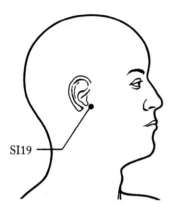
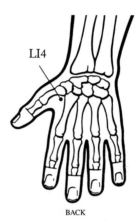

Aromatherapy for Addiction

Aromatherapy can be very helpful in giving up an addiction. Our nasal cavities are in close proximity to our brain, and various smells can open neural pathways, lift moods, give our brains a delightful treat, and promote beneficial states of consciousness. Aromatherapy employs essential oils, the volatile and powerful essences of plants. In addition to being highly aromatic, essential oils offer many healing properties.

Essential oils can be added to a warm bath (use 5 to 10 drops per tubful of water), diluted in vegetable oil for massage (use 40 drops per half cup of oil), or ideally used like smelling salts during the day: just open a bottle and inhale the aroma. Essential oils aren't addicting, but I recommend that you always use a variety of oils, switching from time to

Caution

Essential oils should not be taken internally, applied undiluted to the skin, or put near the eyes. Essential oils should be avoided during pregnancy unless suggested by a professional aromatherapist. Be sure to use pure essential oils and not synthetic smell-alikes.

time to avoid becoming dependent on any one emotional crutch. If you're still using addictive substances but want to begin practicing aromatherapy, use one-half of any recommended dosage.

Though various oils are suggested for various uses, the important thing is that you like the smell. Visit a local supplier of essential oils—such as an herb shop or natural foods store—and smell the testers to get a sense of what each oil does for you.

- **Anise** *(Pimpinella anisum)* improves relaxation and sleep and helps relieve stress caused by overwork. Use it to curb sugar and chocolate cravings.
- **Basil** *(Ocimun basilicum)* is uplifting and helps dispel negative thoughts, indecisiveness, and mental fatigue. In can be used to curb addictive cravings and to aid in withdrawal.
- **Bay** *(Laurus nobilis)* is stimulating and memory enhancing. It helps dispel addictive cravings.
- **Bergamot** *(Citrus bergamia)* helps relieve anxiety, depression, and compulsive behavior. It's effective for treating sugar, food, alcohol, stimulant, and sedative addictions and aids withdrawal.
- **Black pepper** *(Piper nigrum)* stimulates emotions and imparts strength. It can help alleviate the symptoms of nicotine withdrawal.
- **Cardamom** *(Elettaria cardamomum)* is considered invigorating. It helps dispel addictive cravings, especially caffeine.
- **Chamomile, German** *(Matricaria recutita),* is a traditional antidepressant. It calms anxiety and hysteria, helps relieve suppressed anger, and aids sleep. It also helps dispel addictive cravings.
- **Chamomile, Roman** *(Chamaemelum nobile),* is also antidepressant in nature. Use it to treat addictions to sedatives.
- **Clary sage** *(Salvia sclarea)* relieves panic, paranoia, and mental fatigue and improves communication skills. Use it to treat addictions to alcohol and sedatives. It dispels cravings and can be helpful during withdrawal.
- **Eucalyptus** *(Eucalyptus citriodora)* is relaxing. Use it to dispel alcohol cravings.
- **Fennel** *(Foeniculum vulgare)* is stimulating. It helps dispel cravings for alcohol, sugar, and chocolate.

- **Frankincense** *(Boswellia carterii)* enhances spirituality, perception, and states of higher consciousness. It encourages release from the past. Use it for sugar, stimulant, sedative, and other addictive cravings.
- **Geranium** *(Pelargonium graveolens)* is a balancing remedy that relieves anxiety, depression, and stress. Use it for sedative and stimulant addictions. It can be helpful during withdrawal.
- **Grapefruit** *(Citrus paradisi)* is uplifting and aids in inner child work. Use it for stimulant addiction.
- **Helichrysum** *(Helichrysum angustifolium)* lifts depression, stress, and lethargy. Use it for alcohol and tobacco addiction. It's excellent for easing you through the withdrawal period.
- **Jasmine** *(Jasminum officinale, J. grandiflorum)* relieves insomnia, anger, depression, and worry and helps inspire self-confidence. It can dispel addictive cravings.
- **Juniper** *(Juniperus communis)* is recommended for those who are emotionally drained, anxious, and exhausted. Use it to dispel alcohol cravings. It can be helpful during withdrawal.
- **Lavender** *(Lavandula angustifolia)* calms nervousness and relieves exhaustion and depression. It can help dispel addictive cravings, especially for tranquilizers.
- **Lemon** *(Citrus limon)* is an emotionally cleansing antidepressant. It helps relieve irritability and insomnia. It's often recommended as treatment for alcoholism and stimulant addictions.
- **Lime** *(Citrus aurantifolia)* has the same properties as lemon.
- **Marjoram** *(Marjorana hortensis)* relieves emotional instability and irritability. It can be used to relieve loneliness and the pangs of a broken heart. Use it for alcohol and tranquilizer addiction.
- **Neroli** *(Citrus bigardia)* relieves anxiety, depression, fear, and hopelessness. Neroli is a natural tranquilizer and therefore helps reduce addictions to synthetic ones. It relieves shock, imparts strength, and aids sleep.
- **Nutmeg** *(Myristica fragans)* relieves mental exhaustion, stimulates dreams, and lifts depression. It helps dispel addictive cravings and can be used during withdrawal.

- **Orange** *(Citrus sinensis)* relieves stress, hysteria, and tension. Use it for overcoming stimulant addiction.
- **Patchouli** *(Pogostemon cablin)* helps release suppressed emotions. It relieves nervousness and depression and can be used to dispel addictive cravings.
- **Peppermint** *(Mentha piperita)* is stimulating and mentally clearing. Use it for addictions to menthol cigarettes and stimulants.
- **Rose** *(Rosa damascena, R. gallica, R.* spp.) inspires confidence, lifts depression, and helps open the emotional heart to love. It's useful during crises, such as withdrawal. It's especially helpful for treating alcoholism.
- **Rosemary** *(Rosmarinus officinalis)* improves memory and creativity, is stimulating, and enhances perception. It helps dispel addictive cravings.
- **Sandalwood** *(Santalum album)* helps relieve anxiety, depression, and insomnia. It's considered grounding and encourages emotional openness. Use it to treat alcoholism.
- **Spearmint** *(Mentha spicata)* is stimulating and can help you focus. Use it to dispel sugar cravings.
- **Ylang-ylang** *(Canangra odorata)* is sedative in nature. It makes the senses more acute and helps relieve anger, depression, fear, frustration, and jealousy. Use it to dispel addictive cravings, especially to tranquilizers.

Flower Essences for Addiction

Flower essences can help long-suppressed emotions come to the surface and be resolved, which can help cleanse old patterns of addiction. Flower essences can be made by placing fresh picked flowers in springwater for several hours, then collecting and bottling the water. However, flower essences are also easily purchased at quality natural foods stores.

To prepare a personal remedy, take 2 drops of each flower essence you wish to use—you can combine up to six at a time—and place in a clean one-ounce amber-glass dropper bottle. Fill with springwater and add a teaspoon of apple cider vinegar as a preservative. Put

4 drops of the remedy under your tongue four times daily—first thing in the morning, twice during the day, and then again right before bed. The bedtime dose can encourage healing dreams.

There is a tiny amount of alcohol in a "mother" bottle of flower essence, amounting to three or four parts per several hundred parts of water. Once diluted, the alcohol content is infinitesimal. However, if you're struggling with alcoholism and wish to avoid even this tiny bit of alcohol, rather than taking the flower essence orally you can soak in a tubful of water to which 7 drops of flower essence have been added.

- **Agrimony** flower essence is for those who use drugs and alcohol so they can be entertaining or so they can avoid facing their inner self. Beneath a cheerful facade may lie inner turmoil.
- **Angelica** flower essence encourages you to give up alcohol and drugs. It strengthens resolve to face the unknown, allows light into your life, and can help you become realigned with your spiritual path. It's also helpful in getting to the root cause of alcoholism.
- **Arnica** flower essence helps the body deal with the shock of drug and alcohol abuse when the nervous system has experienced damage.
- **Aspen** flower essence is for those who use drugs or alcohol to make themselves less sensitive or to strengthen those who have fear of the unknown.
- **Avocado** flower essence helps eliminate toxins and is especially helpful for treating alcoholism. It's recommended for those who pass through life without goals and who feel foggy.
- **Baby blue eyes** flower essence is for those who abuse substances because they feel the world is too harsh and they are unable to trust in the goodness of life.
- **Black cohosh** flower essence is for those addicted to abusive relationships.
- **Blue China orchid** flower essence helps those addicted and unable to control themselves. It helps strengthen the will and empowers you to feel more in control. It helps relieve feelings of unfulfillment and of being overwhelmed.

- **Bo tree** flower essence helps overcome nicotine addiction.
- **Borage** flower essence gives you the courage to strive for release from addiction.
- **Cayenne** flower essence helps you let go of addictions and promotes quick transformation. It helps you move forward in life.
- **Centaury** flower essence aids the codependent in overcoming victimization and enabling behavior. It also strengthens the willpower of the addict.
- **Chamomile** flower essence calms those going through withdrawal and can sedate hyperactivity.
- **Chaparral** flower essence helps you detoxify on a psychic level.
- **Cherry plum** flower essence helps those who are out of control and governed by their addiction.
- **Chestnut bud** flower essence is for the person who repeats the same mistakes and is in denial. It can help break addictive patterns. It's also useful for the codependent person.
- **Chicory** flower essence is for codependents who allow themselves to be martyred in the process of helping the addict.
- **Chrysanthemum** flower essence is for those using drugs, especially alcohol, to escape pain, loss, and fear of death.
- **Clematis** flower essence is for those who use addictions to escape from their body.
- **Coffee** flower essence is a specific for caffeine addiction, including coffee, chocolate, and cola drinks. It stabilizes the nervous system and calms anxiety.
- **Crab apple** flower essence helps those who feel unclean, guilty, and tired of being addicted.
- **Fairy lantern** flower essence is for those using substances as a form of escape and to be free of adult responsibilities.
- **Gentian** flower essence is for people tormented by worry and negativity. They may use drugs and alcohol to forget their fears. It's also for those with a negative outlook who give up easily.
- **Golden yarrow** flower essence is for those who abuse substances to buffer the effects of social interactions.
- **Gorse** flower essence helps addicts who have a sense of hopelessness from having failed multiple times at giving up their addictions.

- **Golden eardrops** flower essence helps release repressed sadness for those who grew up in alcoholic and dysfunctional families.
- **Impatiens** flower essence is for an irritated nervous system resulting from drug and alcohol abuse.
- **Larch** flower essence can benefit those who don't attempt to give up an addiction for fear of failure.
- **Lavender** flower essence calms nerves exhausted from stimulant use.
- **Milkweed** flower essence can relieve cravings for sedatives.
- **Morning glory** flower essence can be used to ease general withdrawal symptoms. It's recommended as treatment for alcohol, tobacco, caffeine, prescription drug, and stimulant addictions. It tonifies the nervous system, helps relieve nighttime restlessness, and enables you to feel more joyful in greeting the day. Morning glory flower essence can help you break destructive habits, including general compulsive behavior. It also helps rekindle spiritual faith as well as faith in yourself and the future.
- **Oak** flower essence helps those who overeat, overdrink, and abuse chemical substances to make up for their difficult upbringing.
- **Olive** flower essence should be used when the body and mind are depleted from long-term use of stimulants and other drugs.
- **Pennyroyal** flower essence is used as a treatment for alcoholism. It helps repel negative thoughts and enables you to speak out about your true values.
- **Peppermint** flower essence helps you feel more alert without using stimulants.
- **Pink monkey flower** essence is for those who abuse drugs to mask shame and pain.
- **Rosemary** flower essence is for those who use drugs to feel disconnected from their body.
- **Red chestnut** flower essence is for codependents who devote themselves to rescuing others.
- **Red clover** flower essence helps those who have to live or work around addicts cope with the emotional dramas that arise. It can help you remain calm in the face of disaster.
- **Sagebrush** flower essence is for those who cling to illusion. It

Rescue Remedy

Rescue Remedy can be of great help during the withdrawal period, and it can also be used in cases of drug overdose. Rescue Remedy is made from five flower essences: impatiens to instill patience, clematis to promote clear thinking, cherry plum for calm and willpower, rock rose for terror and panic, and star of Bethlehem for emotional trauma. Rescue Remedy is a powerful and safe first-aid remedy for any difficulty in life!

To take Rescue Remedy, simply place 2 drops under the tongue or dilute 2 drops in a glass of water and drink. In times of crisis a drop can be applied to the wrist pulses or forehead.

helps you let go of dysfunctional programming and become more aware of your true identity. It can help you overcome feelings of emptiness during withdrawal.

• **St. John's wort** flower essence can help you be more open to a higher power if addiction has caused you to lose faith. It also calms troubled dreams and relieves fear.

• **Skullcap** flower essence calms nervousness, alleviates deterioration of the nervous system, and strengthens those who are frazzled and preoccupied. It benefits those who have abused caffeine and helps ease their cravings. Skullcap is also beneficial for depression that may occur following drug withdrawal. It helps clear drug residues from the body.

• **Scarlet monkey flower** essence is for those who use drugs to cover feelings of powerlessness and anger.

• **Self-heal** flower essence is used to strengthen the confidence you need to overcome addiction.

• **Star tulip** flower essence is for those who use drugs to create an illusional psychic state.

• **Sunflower** essence is for drug and alcohol abuse resulting from low self-esteem. It helps promote a healthier self-image.

• **Sundew** flower essence helps young people feel more grounded and less indecisive and unfocused. It helps you live in the present.

• **Sweet chestnut** flower essence is for those suffering anguish who have considered suicide and have reached all they can tolerate. It can help them move forward into recovery.

• **Sweet pea** flower essence helps antisocial addicts.

• **Tobacco** flower essence helps you give up the tobacco habit or addictions to drugs that numb feelings of the heart.

• **Walnut** flower essence helps addicts who isolate themselves from others and then abuse substances to cope with the feeling of aloneness.

- **White chestnut** flower essence is for obsessive thoughts and worries, and for the person who abuses substances to calm a racing mind.
- **Wild rose** flower essence is for those who have resigned themselves to addiction and accept it as enslavement.
- **Willow** flower essence helps dissolve emotional bitterness.

Light Therapy

We've known for years that natural light is essential for good health; inadequate light can lead to poor health and can make you more susceptible to developing an addiction. Consider the example reported many years ago in the July 30, 1971, issue of *Science* magazine. Researchers reported that a particular group of rats being studied for alcohol consumption preferred plain water during the week, yet over the weekend went on alcoholic binges. It was discovered that during the weekend the automatic-light timer did not go on, and the rats were being kept in darkness. In the dark they drank; in the light they did not.

Natural light can also aid in detoxification. As reported in a 1988 issue of *Nutrition Health Review,* a team of Austrian psychiatrists and neurologists tested twenty alcoholics suffering from severe withdrawal symptoms. After exposure to bright light for two days, they experienced improvement, better ability to concentrate, better memory, and a reduction in their need for antianxiety medication.

Simply spending an hour a day outdoors is a great way to obtain full-spectrum light. Unless the weather is extremely sunny, do not wear sunglasses, prescription glasses, or even contact lenses so that the full spectrum of light will enter your eyes and pass on to your brain. Doing this before 10 A.M. and after 2 P.M. minimizes your chance of getting a sunburn. If you can't get outside for that long, at least open a door or window so that you'll have some natural light—and fresh air—entering the building, and make an effort to take regular five-minute breaks outdoors.

Color Therapy

The brain is a receptor for color; in fact, the brain often stores experiences according to color-coded memory triggers. How someone reacts to a particular color says something about the memories he or she associates with that color. Studies have shown that addictions can either increase or decrease depending on what colors patients are exposed to. Blue and green were found to be the best colors for those struggling to give up addictions. Blue helps you relax and cools inflammation. Green is balancing and calming. Surround yourself with these colors. Wear clothing in blue and green hues. Visualize breathing in great surges of healing blue and green light. Spend time in green forests and under blue skies whenever possible.

Gem and Crystal Therapy

Gem therapy will seem esoteric to some, yet it's an ancient method of healing and is regaining respect in our current era. Crystals and gems are storehouses of light and energy. Simply holding crystals and gems in each hand during meditation can be grounding, comforting, and healing and can help induce various states of consciousness.

In ancient Europe members of royalty would imbibe their alcohol in amethyst goblets. They believed the amethyst would keep them from becoming inebriated.

Stones should be cleansed before using them for healing work. To cleanse them, bury them in loose sand or earth or place in springwater in either sunlight or moonlight. Passing the crystals through burning sage or artemesia with a prayer of your intention before working with the stones is also a good idea—it helps ground you in your intention for meditation or prayer and gives a sense of sacred space to the ritual.

One simple form of meditation is to sit and hold the crystal and say either to yourself or out loud what your intention is. Concentrate on your purpose. If you like, write your intention on a piece of paper after your ritual; wrap the paper around your crystal and leave it for a few days.

Clear quartz crystal is an ideal tool for prayer and meditation. Other stones to consider are:

- **Green tourmaline** is cleansing.
- **Rhodochrosite** is a beautiful rose color and can help you feel more spiritually connected.
- **Iron pyrite** is sparkly and grounding and helps you keep your feet on the ground.
- **Amethyst** is a traditional preventive for alcoholism.

Try placing healing gems or crystals in the place where your addictive substance is usually kept—the cigarette pack, the pill bottle, the coffee canister, and so on. Hold the stones during meditation or visualization, place them in the bathtub with you, and put them under your pillow when you're sleeping. Keeping them close to you will enable their healing energies to become a part of your energy.

Restructuring Your Relationships

Giving up an addiction is about much more than severing your physical craving for a particular substance. An addiction often arises from psychological needs, fulfills emotional voids, and involves a set pattern of behavior within a circle of your family and friends. What's most important, what's absolutely essential, for kicking an addiction can be boiled down to this: cultivating a good relationship with yourself and with others.

Most of the therapies discussed in this chapter focus on helping you recover self-confidence, emotional stability, and physical independence from addiction. These therapies help you discover or recover a good relationship with yourself. Self-understanding and self-respect are of utmost importance in staying addiction-free. But you also need to take a long, hard look at your relationships with family and friends. Treasure those that are strong and supportive. Improve those that have fallen into disrepair or have been neglected. Try to mend those that bring you self-doubt or those that bring you into situations in which you are likely to relapse into addiction. And turn away from those that cannot be reconciled with your new lifestyle decision. It may be hard, but it must be done.

Addiction keeps you stuck and impairs your ability to grow. Stop postponing. This is the moment! The first step is to admit there is a problem. The second step is to do something about it.

Take your new addiction-free life one day at a time. Tell yourself you're simply not going to indulge for just this one day. Tomorrow, tell yourself the same thing. By the third day, you have already come a long way. You deserve to be happy and free. Best wishes to all of you who are brave enough to take action!

PART TWO

Healing Begins

3

Like a Kid in
a Candy Store
Sugar Addictions

Sugar is not only the most prevalent addiction in our society, but it's also the least recognized and one of the hardest to kick. You may think, *What's this—sugar? An addiction?* The answer is a resounding yes! Think about it—have you ever seen a kid freak out in the vegetable aisle? And have you ever had an overwhelming, makes-your-mouth-water, not-to-be-denied craving for, say, a turnip? Doesn't quite inspire the same feelings of passion that so many of us—especially women—have for chocolate, does it?

Sugar, like a drug, makes the body feel good, and when that feeling passes, the body craves more. Yet almost no one calls sugar an addictive substance. What's truly frightening about it is that sugar is found in practically every food product on the grocery store shelf. Are we a society of unknowing addicts? Perhaps.

Sweet History

Sugar is derived from sugarcane *(Saccharum officinarum)* and sugar beet *(Beta vulgaris).*

Sugarcane is native to the islands of the southeast Pacific. The Pacific Islanders were intrepid travelers, and where they went, so too did sugarcane. By 3000 B.C. India was processing a form of sugar from sugarcane; they called it *gaura*. When Persians invaded India in 510 B.C., they were enraptured by the "reed which gives honey without bees." Sugar and sugarcane soon migrated to Arab countries and eventually to Europe; the Crusaders carried this "new spice" home with them. Centuries later Christopher Columbus brought sugarcane plants with him to the Caribbean. Sugarcane plantations, manned by slave labor, quickly spread across the islands.

Sugar beets, which are native to Eurasia, were grown as a sweet vegetable by many ancient cultures, including the Indians, Egyptians, Greeks, Romans, and Chinese. Once identified as a source of sugar, sugar beets increased rapidly in popularity. By 1889 sugar beets had replaced sugarcane as the main European sugar source.

Sugar was so precious in past ages that it was used only in small amounts to flavor medicines. And it was expensive—in the early fourteenth century sugar sold for two shillings a pound in London. Today this would be about a hundred dollars a kilo, or almost fifty dollars a pound. One hundred years ago the average American ate about four pounds of sugar a year. Now that number has risen to about 150 pounds per person per year. That adds up to five tons in a lifetime!

White sugar as we know it first became available in 1812, when a chemist found a way to make "chemically pure" sugar, defined as 99.5 percent sucrose.

To make white sugar, sugarcane is first crushed, or sugar beets are first sliced, and infused in hot water. The cane or beets are then fed through rollers to extract their juice. The juice is filtered through charred animal bones to remove impurities, then boiled to allow excess water to evaporate, and then seeded with sugar crystals to encourage crystallization. After crystallization the sugar is spun in high-speed machines, similar to clothes dryers, which separate the sugar from the syrup.

A Refined Dependency

In our society we are born and bred to be sugar addicts. Unlike other highly addictive substances—cocaine, heroin, prescription drugs—which can be difficult to procure, finding food products *without* sugar can be a challenge. By the time most people have their first experience with alcohol, tobacco, or drugs, they've been sugar addicts for years.

Nature most likely planned us to be attracted to the nutrients available in sweet foods. For example, our first food, mother's milk, is naturally sweet. However, the process of refining—which is as complex as that for getting heroin from poppies and cocaine from coca leaves—removes all the accompanying nutrients and fiber from the original plant material. Only the sucrose is kept. Because sugar is so refined, it doesn't require much processing by the body and passes almost directly into the intestines and bloodstream—just like a drug. And like a drug, sugar can be habit forming. If you don't think you're addicted, just try to go a couple of weeks without it!

> **Eastern Perspectives on Sugar**
>
> In traditional Chinese medicine sugar cravings are seen as a desire for "the mother energy" or a need for comfort and security.

Sugar addiction is, in part, a by-product of sugar's purity—the body is not suited to accommodate this level of refinement. Simple sugars—found in white table sugar, corn syrup, fructose, honey, white flour, or any other super-refined carbohydrate—are refined to the point that digestion is practically superfluous. When you consume simple sugars, they are passed quickly into the bloodstream. Blood sugar levels skyrocket, and you experience a lift in energy. But that feeling of increased energy and mental alertness is very temporary. As most of us can confirm, sugar highs lead to sugar crashes. And when that buzz wears off, the body cries out for more sugar.

Sugar is also an antidepressant of sorts. Consumption of sugar triggers the release of the brain chemical serotonin, which elevates mood and alleviates depression. Sugar cravings are often a misguided attempt by the body to increase serotonin levels in the system and thus elevate mood. Sugar cravings can also be caused by low endorphin levels, hypoglycemia, endocrine imbalances, candida, and nutritional deficiencies.

Studies in prisons indicate that violence is remarkably reduced when sugar and refined carbohydrates are eliminated from the diet.

Those suffering from sugar addiction often experience irritability, headaches, mood swings, and insomnia. Signs of sugar withdrawal include restlessness, nervousness, headache, and depression.

The Real Scoop on Sugar

It's an undisputed fact that sugar contributes to dental cavities. Sugar interacts with bacteria in the mouth to produce acids that make holes in the teeth enamel. Sugar also contributes to plaque accumulation. Knowing this, do we cut back on our sugar consumption? No. We simply put fluoride in our drinking water and train more dentists.

But sugar has a great many more ill effects on the human body. Sugar stands accused of causing both hypoglycemia and diabetes. It has been linked to numerous mental disorders, including depression, hyperactivity, obsessive-compulsive disorders, and phobias. It weakens the immune system, encourages the growth of infections, and lowers the production of antibodies. It overtaxes the spleen, pancreas, and small intestines. Overconsumption of sugar contributes to the development of allergies, anemia, arthritis, cancer, Crohn's disease, gout, headaches, heart disease, herpes, hyperactivity, impotence, obesity, osteoporosis, PMS, and yeast infections.

Sugar is often called an antinutrient. Overconsumption of simple sugars causes the body to use up its supplies of calcium, potassium, thiamin, and chromium. And all sugars, even natural ones, appear to compete with vitamin C for transportation into white blood cells. Without adequate amounts of vitamin C, the immune system becomes severely compromised.

The -Ose Cousins

Check the ingredients list on some prepared foods in your refrigerator and cabinets. You just might be surprised at how much sugar is in them. Don't see "sugar" listed? Look for its "-ose" cousins: fructose, dextrose, sucrose, maltose, et cetera. They may hide behind high-tech chemical names, but at heart they're all sugar.

The -ose cousins come in a range of molecular complexity. Monosaccharides, or simple sugars, are quickly digested and passed on almost directly to the bloodstream. Disaccharides are slightly more complex; they must be broken down by enzymes before they can be fully digested. Polysaccharides are even more complex; these are the sugars you find naturally occurring in whole grains and starches. The more complex a sugar is, the more slowly it's digested, and the less startling the effect it has on your blood sugar levels.

Some of the more common -ose cousins you're likely to come across include:

- **Dextrose** is made from corn, sugarcane, or sugar beets. It's a highly refined monosaccharide and is thus very quickly absorbed.
- **Fructose,** also known as levulose, occurs naturally in fruits, many plants, and honey. For commercial purposes it's derived from corn, sugarcane, or sugar beets. Although it's more slowly absorbed than white sugar (sucrose),

Sugar and Diabetes

The link between sugar consumption and diabetes was recognized as long ago as 1929, when Sir Frederick Banting observed that Panamanian sugar plantation owners, who consumed refined sugar, had a much higher incidence of diabetes than their workers, who ate only unrefined cane sugar.

When simple sugars are ingested, they raise blood glucose levels. The pancreas responds by releasing insulin, which stabilizes the blood sugar levels. Over time, if simple sugars are overconsumed, the pancreas becomes overly sensitive to sugar, and insulin secretion becomes excessive, causing a persistent hypoglycemic state. If this pattern continues, the pancreas becomes overworked and ceases to be a reliable source of insulin; the body suffers from elevated blood sugar levels and can develop Type 2 diabetes. The incidence of adult-onset diabetes in the United States has increased proportionately to the increase in sugar consumption. Diabetes is now the seventh leading cause of death in the United States.

it's still a highly refined simple sugar. It's slightly sweeter than white sugar.

- **Glucose** is the same sugar our bodies use for energy; it's also found in many fruits, vegetables, and grains. Glucose is stored by the liver in the form of glycogen and released when a burst of energy is needed. It's a monosaccharide, or simple sugar, and is absorbed into the bloodstream almost immediately. When glucose is derived from foods such as legumes and whole grains, it's metabolized more slowly and is easier on the body.

- **Lactose** is a disaccharide composed of glucose and galactose. Found in the milk of mammalian mothers, it's only slightly sweet.

- **Maltose.** Also known as malt sugar, maltose is found in barley and rice syrups. As a disaccharide, or complex sugar, it takes longer to digest, which is desirable: it keeps blood sugar levels from skyrocketing. It's made by the fermentation of starches by enzymes or yeast.

- **Sucrose** is composed mainly of glucose and fructose. It comprises 99.5 percent of common white table sugar. A simple sugar, it's speedily absorbed by the body.

What About Artificial Sweeteners?

Without sugar substitutes we'd have no one-calorie soda and no sugar-free ice cream. Artificial sweeteners offer that sweet taste with few or no calories; as the labels say, they are indeed nonnutritive. But they're also potentially among the most toxic food additives in the grocery store today. Studies have linked the two most common artificial sweeteners, aspartame and saccharin, to cancer development in mice and rats. Saccharin is synthesized from petrochemicals. Aspartame produces methanol—a volatile, flammable, poisonous liquid alcohol—in the digestive tract. Is this what you want to put in your body? You might be better off with sugar!

All the Sugar in the World

There are myriad sugar manifestations and simulations. Below you'll find descriptions of the most common sugars and sugar substitutes you're likely to find in a grocery or natural foods store. Don't think, though, that because a sweetener is all-natural it's also better for you than white sugar. Most alternatives to white table sugar are comprised almost completely of simple sugars and can affect your body to almost the same

degree as can straight sucrose. Read the
descriptions carefully. If you're looking for
alternatives to white table sugar, seek out
those that are not stripped of their nutrients,
that are absorbed by the body more slowly
than white sugar, and that are not composed solely of simple sugars.

> Mosquitoes are more attracted to people who eat lots of sugar.

- **Agave** is derived from the blue agave plant. It's absorbed by the
  body more slowly than white table sugar; it's rich in natural
  fructose and nutrients such as calcium, iron, magnesium, and
  potassium.
- **Amasake** is made from rice that has
  been inoculated with koji, the same
  aspergillus culture used to make miso.
  During fermentation, the rice starches
  are converted to sugar, making them
  sweet and easy to digest. Amasake is
  about 21 percent simple sugars, namely
  glucose and maltose. It also contains
  some carbohydrates, iron, potassium, and B vitamins.

> Diabetics and hypoglycemics should avoid all concentrated sweeteners except under the advice of a qualified health care professional.

- **Aspartame** is made by combining two amino acids, aspartic acid
  and phenylalanine. It's currently found in more than three thousand food products. Aspartame contains only about four calories
  per gram and is 180 to 200 times sweeter than white sugar, so
  very little is needed. Aspartame can cause headaches, dizziness,
  numbness, cramps, abdominal pain, depression, and, in certain
  individuals, seizures. Although laboratory studies show that it
  can cause brain tumors in animals, and there is concern that it
  can cause mental retardation in unborn babies, aspartame is
  approved as a sweetener. When it's heated, the methanol con-
  tained in aspartame breaks down into carcinogenic formalde-
  hyde. For those rare people who suffer from phenylketonuria,
  consuming aspartame can cause irreversible mental retardation.
  There have been more complaints about aspartame to the Food
  and Drug Administration (FDA) than any other food additive
  in the FDA's history.

- **Barley, rye, and wheat malts.** Barley malt syrup is a traditional sugar substitute. It's made from soaked, sprouted, or dried barley that has been cooked with water to make a sweet dark syrup. It can ferment if stored longer than a year. Because it's aborbed more slowly than sugar, it has a less extreme effect on blood sugar levels. The sweetness in barley malt syrup derives from maltose and glucose; it's about 40 percent complex carbohydrates and 3 percent protein. Rye and wheat malts are new to the sugar substitute field. They have similar properties to barley malt.

- **Brown sugar** is white sugar with a small amount of molasses added back in. It's about 93.8 percent sucrose and has very small amounts of calcium, iron, and potassium.

- **Cane sugar.** Unrefined cane sugar (also known as granulated cane juice) is simply sugarcane with its water content removed. It's processed mechanically rather than with chemicals. About 85 percent sucrose, it has a fuller, more rounded flavor than white table sugar. It contains all of the minerals naturally occurring in sugarcane as well as some of the trace mineral chromium, B vitamins, and amino acids, which can all help curb sugar cravings.

- **Carob** tastes similar to chocolate but does not contain any caffeine. Without any additives, it's about 46 percent sugars. It also contains some protein, B vitamins, and potassium.

- **Corn syrup.** Corn starch with all its nutrients chemically removed except the starch makes corn syrup. It's absorbed very quickly by the body. It contains up to 70 percent simple sugars (mostly glucose) as well as some complex carbohydrates. It's somewhat less sweet than white table sugar. Many people are allergic to corn, and thus to corn syrup as well.

- **Date sugar** is made of dehydrated ground dates. It contains sucrose, glucose, fructose, complex carbohydrates, and all the nutrients

Unrefined cane sugar does not cause tooth decay. In a study conducted in 1937 at the University of Witwatersrand in South Africa, scientists placed thirty-two extracted teeth in water sweetened with refined sugar. After eight weeks fifteen of the teeth had developed cavities. When the same study was done on teeth submerged in unrefined cane juice, only three teeth developed cavities.

found in dates. It's about equal in sweetness to regular sugar.

- **Fruit juice.** Fruit juice concentrates are usually derived from grapes, peaches, pears, and pineapples. They're usually about 68 percent simple sugars, mainly sucrose and fructose.

- **Honey** is made from flowers by the grace of bees. Flower nectar is rich in sucrose, and the bees transform this product with their stomach enzymes into honey. Bees work hard for this commodity: the average bee produces half a teaspoon of honey in its entire lifetime. Honey contains trace amounts of vitamins, minerals, and enzymes. The darker honeys are richer in minerals. Honey contains fructose, sucrose, and glucose. Like white sugar, it's quickly absorbed into the bloodstream. However, it's sweeter than sugar, so less of it can be used. Buy raw unfiltered honey, because heat processing can destroy honey's valuable yet delicate enzymes.

- **Mannitol** is sugar alcohol that is slightly less sweet than white table sugar. Natural mannitol is derived from plants, most commonly seaweed, but commercial-grade mannitol is derived from sugar.

- **Maple syrup** is derived from the sap of sugar maple trees. It takes about forty gallons of sap from a maple tree to produce just one gallon of maple syrup. Maple syrup is about 65 percent sucrose; it also contains some B vitamins as well as calcium and potassium. The lighter syrups, which are given the higher grade of A, have lesser amounts of minerals than do the darker, lower—and less expensive—grades such as B and C. If maple

> When sugarcane is cut, it's composed of only about 10 to 14 percent sucrose. After being refined, it's 99.5 percent sucrose.

> Commercial fruit juice concentrates made from grapes can have an especially high amount of pesticide residues.

> Don't give honey to children under the age of two. Honey can contain tiny amounts of botulism spores, which are not a danger for adults but can cause problems for the still-developing digestive systems of very young children.

Mannitol should not be given to children, as it can give them diarrhea. It has also been implicated in gastrointestinal and kidney disturbances in adults.

syrup isn't labeled PURE MAPLE SYRUP, it may be cut with corn syrup. Maple sugar is made from the syrup.

• **Molasses.** As a by-product of sugar manufacture, molasses contains the nutrients that are removed from white table sugar. It's 50 to 70 percent simple sugars, but it also contains some B vitamins, iron, and calcium. Blackstrap molasses is less refined and higher in nutrients than the lighter varieties. Look for unsulfured varieties; sulfur dioxide is sometimes used as a molasses preservative and bleaching agent, and it destroys vitamins A and B, is highly irritating to the body, and can cause allergic reactions for sensitive people.

• **Raw sugar** is white table sugar just before the molasses has been extracted. It's about 96 percent sucrose and still retains a trace amount of minerals.

• **Rice syrup** is often made from cooked rice and sprouted barley. It has a milder flavor than straight barley malt. Of all the sweeteners, it's the one highest in protein and does contain some B vitamins and potassium, especially if made from brown rather than white rice. Brown rice syrup contains maltose, glucose, and complex carbohydrates. It has a pleasant butterscotch-like flavor.

• **Saccharin** is manufactured from petroleum and toluene. It's severely sweet and calorie-free. Research done with rats has linked saccharin to bladder cancer and kidney damage. In 1977 the FDA wanted to ban it, but such was the outcry from sugar-crazed consumers that saccharin is now permitted, although warning labels must be posted on its packages.

• **Sorbitol** is a sugar alcohol derived from glucose and dextrose. Like mannitol, it's made from corn and is about 60 percent as sweet as sugar. Since it's absorbed slowly, it's often used as a sweetener by diabetics. It's unlikely to cause tooth decay, though some people have complained of diarrhea from its use. There has also been some suspicion that sorbitol can cause cataracts.

• **Sorghum** is the concentrated juice of a plant called sweet sorghum *(Horcus sorghum saccara),* a relative of millet. It's about 65 percent sucrose with some mineral content. It has a taste slightly lighter than that of molasses.

In addition to being a sweetener, stevia is traditionally used as a wound healer, tonic, energizer, and digestive aid.

- **Stevia** is a perennial shrub with a long history of use in South America as a sweetener. One leaf is enough to sweeten a cup of tea yet contains less than one-tenth of a calorie. Stevia contains 20 percent stevioside, a glycoside that is about two hundred times sweeter than sugar. Though further studies are being conducted, it seems not to have adverse effects for those with diabetes, hypoglycemia, or candida.
- **Turbinado sugar** is sugarcane or sugar beets at an intermediate stage between raw sugar and refined sugar. It's about 95 percent sucrose.
- **White sugar.** This is the common table sugar we're accustomed to. White sugar is 99.5 percent sucrose. All of its nutrients are removed in processing and bleaching. It's derived from either sugar beets or sugarcane, which are usually grown with large amounts of chemical fertilizers and pesticides and deplete the soil quickly. Sugar contains calories but no vitamins or minerals, and as you've read earlier it can actually deplete the body of nutrients.
- **Xylitol** is derived from xylan, a compound found in birchwood pulp, pecan shells, straw, and corncobs. It has the same sweetness as sucrose but doesn't cause cavities and may even neutralize acids in the mouth that decay the teeth. There's some controversy as to whether or not xylitol irritates the bladder.

Chocolate: Sugar Addiction and Then Some

Chocolate comes from the seed of the cacao plant *(Theobroma cacao),* which is native to the American Tropics. Cacao goes by various names, including *chocolate, cocoa, cacaotier,* and *devil's food.* The common *chocolate* derives from the Aztec word for the cacao plant, *chócolatl.*

The seed of the cacao plant is composed of about 2.5 percent

Cacao Facts

- Cacao beans were once used as a currency in the Yucatán.
- *Theobroma*, the genus name given to cacao by the Swedish botanist Linnaeus, translates as "food of the gods."
- Cacao is high in magnesium, so if you have strong chocolate cravings, your body may be trying to let you know that supplementation is in order.

naturally occurring sugars (sucrose and dextrose), 3 percent theobromine, a small amount of caffeine, and 40 to 60 percent fat. The combination of theobromine and caffeine makes chocolate a potent stimulant. Theobromine opens the coronary artery, increasing blood flow to the heart and improving circulation. Caffeine, as discussed in chapter 4, stimulates the nervous system, masking fatigue and increasing energy levels. In fact, chocolate bars were issued to U.S. armed forces during World War II as "fighting food"; it was believed that the chocolate would help them stay awake and alert.

Cacao is naturally bitter to the taste. Most commercial chocolate today, however, has a low cacao content and high levels of sugar and hydrogenated oil. Sugar, as I have discussed, is an addictive substance that stimulates highs in both energy and mood. Chocolate's fats elevate levels of endorphins and enkephalins, which lift mood and soothe frazzled nerves, as well as of a chemical called phenylethylamine. Phenylethylamine is an addictive, mood-elevating, amphetamine-like stimulant. It's used by the brain to make norepinephrine, which slows the breakdown of endorphins and enkephalines. Psychiatrists have theorized that those who binge on chocolate may have an inability to regulate natural body levels of phenylethylamine.

Since it contains both sugar and caffeine, chocolate is a highly addictive substance. It can aggravate chronic states of insomnia, anxiety, and irritability and contribute to acne, cavities, depression, heartburn, heart disease, herpes, irritable bowel, kidney stones, migraines, obesity, and shingles. Withdrawal can cause headaches and intense cravings.

Behavior Therapy

Start by keeping a food journal. Write down everything you eat and drink, from the juice you drink at breakfast to the bite of chocolate you have to help you through the afternoon at work to the pasta and bread you eat for dinner. Tracking your eating habits can help you be more aware of just how much sugar—in the form of white sugar and simple carbohydrates—you're consuming.

Read labels when you're shopping. You'll likely be surprised at how much sugar (of many different varieties) is in the food you're accustomed to eating.

Cut back on your sugar intake gradually so you don't shock your system. Begin by banishing high-sugar sweets from your home. Start eating more whole grains and fewer pastas and breads made from white flour. When you have a sugar craving in the afternoon, eat a banana or an apple. Use seven-grain bread instead of white. Substitute natural sugars for refined white table sugar.

At first, avoiding foods high in simple sugars, such as chocolate, ice cream, and white bread, can be difficult. You may be a bit irritable, suffer from mood swings, and feel mentally sluggish, and you may have to battle with yourself not to give in to your sugar cravings. In just a few weeks, however, you'll find that saying no to sweets is second nature. You'll feel energized, alert, and healthier, and you will no longer suffer from sugar cravings. Eating less sugar will improve your physical and emotional health. And the more you improve the condition of your body and mind, the less you'll crave sugar.

Nutritional Therapy

To keep your blood sugar levels stable and to minimize sugar cravings, eat foods rich in protein and B vitamins. To break the sugar habit, avoid refined carbohydrates such as white bread, white rice, and pasta; eat more complex carbohydrates such as oatmeal, brown rice, and millet. Eat less salt, and fewer dairy products; they'll cause you to crave something sweet later.

Slow down and savor the natural sweetness in food, noticing the "full" taste rather than the "hollow," empty-of-nutrients sweetness. Chew all your food slowly and thoroughly. Be present with what you're eating. Enjoy herbal teas without sweeteners. On occasion, make desserts out of the more suitable sweeteners listed on pages 111–11.

Craving sweets can be an indication that the body needs more protein. Nuts can be a good snack alternative.

When you have sugar cravings, eat sweet foods that are more nourishing than sugary sweets, such as beets, carrots, Jerusalem artichokes, parsnips, sweet potatoes, winter squash, and corn. If you really need a fix, try slowly eating some fresh fruit or figs.

Supplement Therapy

There's a variety of supplements you can take that will help ease you through the withdrawal period and repair some of the damage sugar has done to your health.

SUPPLEMENT	DOSAGE	COMMENTS
B-complex vitamins	25–100 mg	Will help you overcome sugar cravings.
Calcium-magnesium	1,000 mg calcium plus 500 mg magnesium daily	Will help you overcome sugar cravings. Supplements can help you keep your cool during the sugar withdrawal period.
Vitamin C	3,000 mg daily	Antioxidant; also essential for tissue repair.
Zinc	15–25 mg daily	Antioxidant; also essential for tissue repair.
Chromium	200 mcg up to five times daily	Stabilizes blood sugar levels, helps insulin work more efficiently, and keeps your mind off sweets. Decrease this dosage as you can.
L-glutamine	500 mg four times daily	Helps satisfy the body's craving for sugar. Take your dosages between meals for maxium effect.
L-glycine	500 mg twice daily	Has a calming effect on the mind and, in the recommended dosages, can be energizing. Take your dosages between meals for maximum effect.

Spirulina, blue-green algae, and chlorella supplements can help deter sugar cravings by providing protein and nourishing complex carbohydrates. You can usually buy these supplements in natural food sstores; follow the dosage instruction on the package.

Herbal Therapy

Gymnema is a superb sugar buster. Gymnema prevents the taste buds from being activated by sugar and actually blocks sugar from being absorbed during digestion. The molecular arrangement of gymnema is very similar to that of glucose; it adheres to the sensors in the taste buds where sugar would be tasted. The tissue structure in the intestines is similar to that of the taste buds; gymnema fills the receptor sites there as well so that sugar is not absorbed. And when gymnema is ingested, it decreases the desire to eat sweet foods. To help kick your sugar habit, take 2 gymnema capsules three times daily. As your sugar cravings diminish, decrease the dosage.

To stave off a strong sugar craving, take a dose of herbal bitters—about 1 dropperful of tincture—on your tongue. You can find herbal bitters at most natural foods stores and herb shops.

Herbal Therapy for Chocolate Cravings

If you're craving chocolate, try drinking tea made from anise, fennel, and licorice root. These herbs are nutritive and contain natural sugars that stabilize blood sugar levels, thus helping diminish the cravings for sweets. You can also do inhalations of aromatic essential oils, which will give your brain a dose of something pleasurable without indulging in anything addictive. Several essential oils are particularly helpful in staving off chocolate cravings:

- **Anise** smells sweet and is naturally calming.
- **Cardamom** is naturally spicy and invigorating—a great combination for chocolate lovers.
- **Cinnamon** smells sweet, calms the nerves, and invigorates the senses.
- **Clove** smells spicy and reduces mental fatigue and nervousness.

- **Fennel** smells sweet and stimulating, and reduces cravings for sweets.
- **Nutmeg** is stimulating and promotes alertness.
- **Rose** promotes feelings of love and emotional openness, lifts depression, and gives comfort during times of sorrow.
- **Vanilla** is sweet and helps diminish pent-up frustrations.

Sugar Substitutes

Cutting refined sugar from your diet doesn't mean that there'll be no sweetness in your life. Just substitute natural sweeteners, and use them in moderation. Those sweeteners followed by an asterisk (*) have more complex components, have a slower effect on blood sugar, and thus should be preferred.

For every cup of white sugar called for in a recipe, substitute one of the items on the following chart.

NATURAL SWEETENER	AMOUNT TO SUBSTITUTE FOR 1 CUP SUGAR	COMMENTS
Agave syrup*	Use in equal amounts to sugar called for.	Reduce any liquids called for in recipe by one-half to one-third.
Amasake*	1½ cups	Reduce any liquids called for in recipe by one-half
Barley malt syrup*	1⅓ cups	Reduce any liquids called for in recipe by one-fourth. Adding ¼ tsp. baking soda for every cup barley malt used will help baked goods rise.
Cane sugar, unrefined*	Use in equal amounts to sugar called for.	
Date sugar*	⅔–1 cup	Burns easily, so cook with care.
Fruit juice concentrate	⅔ cup	Reduce any liquids called for in recipe by one-third. Add ¼ tsp. baking soda for every cup fruit sweetener.
Granulated fruit sweetener	1¼ cups	Avoid baking at higher than 350 degrees..

NATURAL SWEETENER	AMOUNT TO SUBSTITUTE FOR 1 CUP SUGAR	COMMENTS
Fructose	$1/2$–$2/3$ cup	
Honey*	$1/2$ cup	Reduce any liquids called for in recipe by one-eighth. Reduce oven temperature by 25 degrees and cook things a bit longer.
Maple syrup*	$3/4$ cup	Reduce any liquid called for in recipe by a little less than one-fourth (by 3 tablespoons for every cup). Add $1/4$ tsp. baking soda for every cup maple syrup used.
Molasses*	$1/2$ cup	Reduce any liquids called for in recipe by one-fourth.
Rice syrup*	$1^{1}/3$ cups	Reduce any liquids called for in recipe by one-fourth. If you're baking, add $1/4$ tsp. baking soda for every cup rice syrup to help product rise.
Sorghum	$1/2$ cup	Reduce any liquids called for in recipe by one-fourth.
Stevia*	1 tsp.	Increase any liquids in recipe by one-eighth. Wow!

4

The Java Jones
Giving Up Caffeine

Who doesn't start the day with a steaming cup of java? Or do you prefer English breakfast tea with sugar and milk? Isn't that what morning is all about? Unfortunately, for most people the answer is yes. And what a way to start your day! It's simply rude and unhealthy for your body to go from rest and fasting overnight to drinking a stimulant first thing in the morning. Most people at least warm up their cars on a cold morning; we should do more to respect our body's natural rhythms. Add the caffeine present in chocolate and soft drinks to your daily coffee or tea tally and you may well find that you consume more caffeine than you think.

If the thought of going without your ritual morning mug of joe (or jane) inspires sheer panic, you can be sure that you're addicted. But your symptoms may be more subtle. Perhaps you ran late one morning, had to zoom in to work without the benefit of caffeine, and ended up with a shrieking headache. Or maybe you skipped your afternoon cup because a meeting ran overtime and discovered that without your cola or latté you couldn't make it through the afternoon. But if you're like most people who drink coffee or tea regularly, you already know that you need a certain minimum amount of caffeine to get through the day—and that's addiction!

If you are addicted, you're not alone. Addiction to caffeine is widespread in our workaholic society. It makes us ignore the body's requests for some downtime and allows us to drive ourselves ever more frantically. When we continue to rely on stimulants for energy, we never get to check in with how we really feel. Are we sleeping well? Eating well? Giving our bodies the raw materials they need to sustain our energy levels throughout the day? (See chapter 10 to learn how to increase your energy.)

Although most of us ingest caffeine on a regular basis, it is in fact a drug—and one with profound effects on the human body. Caffeine is a naturally occurring alkaloid found in a number of leaves, seeds, and fruits such as coffee, tea, cola nuts, guarana, and cocoa beans. Caffeine can also be produced synthetically and added to food or drug products. Many soft drinks contain this common stimulant—some, such as Jolt, tout their high caffeine content—and these days you can even buy caffeinated springwater. Caffeine stimulates the nervous system directly, masking fatigue and increasing energy levels. It also increases heart and breathing rates as well as endocrine activity. Just a few minutes after caffeine is ingested, it's already in your bloodstream and making the rounds of your body.

Product	Caffeine Content (per 6-ounce serving)
Drip coffee	70–160 mg
Instant coffee	95 mg
Espresso	50–130 mg
Decaffeinated coffee	5 mg
Cola	45 mg
Chocolate bar	25 mg
Black tea	35 mg
Decaffeinated black tea	4 mg
Green tea	6–30 mg
Oolong tea	10–45 mg

The impact of caffeine on the body can be positive, neutral, or negative, depending largely on how much is being consumed and how often. In small amounts caffeine can actually improve athletic performance by temporarily increasing muscle endurance and strength. Caffeine can also help us think more clearly and feel more alert, but this effect is short lived: we quickly build up tolerance with regular use. Sleep studies have shown that brain waves are more rapid after caffeine intake, with fewer delta waves—the ones that signal the body is recuperating and repairing itself—as well as less dream time. In people who are particularly caffeine sensitive, caffeine can trigger migraine headaches, but for others taking caffeine at the onset can actually avert a migraine, especially when taken as a tablespoon of lemon juice mixed in with a cup of tea or coffee.

Caffeine is used in certain medicines to intensify the effects of other substances and promote a sense of well-being. It also helps to increase the pain-relieving actions of analgesics. Caffeine can alter the effects of both prescription and nonprescription drugs in ways that are unpredictable. Be aware that caffeine makes an appearance in many over-the-counter medications, including NoDoz, Anacin, Midol, Dexatrim, Excedrin, Vanquish, Aqua-Ban, and Dietac.

Caffeine can actually be fatal in high doses: 10 grams, the equivalent of 100 cups of coffee or 167 cups of black tea. But staying under the 10-gram-a-day limit does not mean that heavy caffeine consumption is safe. Researchers now agree that excessive caffeine intake—more than 500 milligrams per day for an adult, or any regular amount of consumption for children—is definitely dangerous. Numerous studies have documented caffeine's many adverse effects.

Caffeinism is the term for caffeine addiction. It can cause anxiety, depression, insomnia, muscle tension, headaches, heart palpitations, heartburn, irritability, and digestive distress.

Too much caffeine can cause a rapid or irregular heart rate, dehydration, nausea, vomiting, anxiety, tremors, depression, and insomnia. Heavy caffeine use also has an impact on fibrocystic breast disease, cardiovascular disease, birth defects, and reproductive problems. But how much is too much?

There is no simple answer to this question, but if you're feeling caffeine's most common negative effects—anxiety, nervousness, and insomnia—and you consume any caffeinated substances on a regular basis, perhaps it's time to cut back. The healthiest relationship to have with caffeine is one in which you remain in control. Read on for ways to regain balance and energize your body naturally.

Coffee

Coffee break, coffeehouse, coffee cake—our culture is obsessed with coffee. Even those who feel a religious or moral motivation to avoid alcohol and tobacco often see nothing wrong with drinking coffee. Coffee is the most widely used herb in America. Nowadays Americans consume about one-third of the world's coffee production, with the average American drinking twenty-eight gallons a year. The fact that coffee is often combined with sugar compounds the addiction. And it's no mystery why many of us fall prey to coffee's seductive promise of higher energy and clearer thought. Did you ever notice how so many places of employment (even some health foods stores) offer free coffee to employees? Just keep those workers cranking!

Modern-day office warriors participate in a new form of an ancient tradition when they stop by Starbucks on their way to work. During prehistoric times coffee beans in their red unroasted form were eaten in East Africa to fortify hunters before tribal wars. Similarly, in ninth-century Ethiopia coffee was considered a food; crushed coffee beans were

Eastern Perspectives on Coffee

In traditional Chinese medicine coffee is considered beneficial when used appropriately. It's said to liberate essential reserves of energy, also known as essence or jing; caffeine transforms jing into chi, or life force, which energizes and activates the body. Overuse can exhaust your natural reserves of jing, however; you temporarily feel more energized but in the long run can become depleted. Coffee is considered energetically bitter, pungent, cold-surface relieving, and warm. While initially heating, its long-term effect is more cooling. Those with yang deficiencies (known as a damp condition, characterized by fluid retention and a feeling of fullness in the abdomen) will tolerate coffee better than those considered yin deficient (generally dry and lacking moisture). Those with overly hot constitutions as well as those who are weak or frail should avoid coffee.

Eating an apple will dispel coffee breath.

molded with fat into balls and consumed by nomadic people. This mixture was also consumed before going to war with neighboring tribes to bolster courage.

The practice of drinking coffee began about a thousand years ago in the region now known as Ethiopia, formerly called Caffa. According to legend, when an Arab mullah encountered a goat herder named Galdi who had a flock of frolicking goats, he questioned Galdi about their excited behavior. The goat herder pointed out the bush they had been grazing upon. When the mullah tried some of the beans, he, too, felt excited. He brought some coffee berries back to the monastery, where they were particularly enjoyed by the mullahs performing all-night prayer vigils.

Around A.D. 1500 spice traders brought coffee into Italy; its use spread throughout Europe during the next few centuries. The first coffeehouse opened in London in 1625 and in Boston in 1670. The Catholic Church tried to ban coffee in the seventeenth century, but Pope Clement VIII consumed his fair share and brought acceptance to the practice. Soon after, cappuccino was developed as a purported remedy for bubonic plague.

For many years Arabs held the monopoly in coffee import through the port of Mocha; no one was allowed to export the plant or unroasted seeds. In 1690 the Dutch managed to smuggle out coffee seedlings, which were then planted in Java. By the early seventeenth century coffee trees were being planted in Jamaica and Martinique, then Central America and Brazil.

After tea was dumped in Boston Harbor in 1773, coffee drinking increased among the colonists. Many of the feelings that fueled the American Revolution took root in the coffeehouses that sprang up in cities, giving people a place to gather and voice their opinions. Not long after, coffee replaced beer as the main morning beverage.

Coffee *(Coffea arabica, C. robusta, C. liberica)* is a member of the Rubiaceae family and also goes by such names as Arabian coffee, devil's brew, café, and java. What we actually drink is a "tea" made from coffee. The part of the plant that brings us this brew is the kernel of a ripe dried seed—or, more accurately, of a coffee berry. These berries are red and fleshy with a thin parchment covering that must be removed before roasting. Roasting makes the beans less acidic and improves their aroma and flavor.

As a medicinal plant, coffee is an antioxidant, antiemetic, antinarcotic, appetite suppressant, bronchial dilator, cardiac stimulant, cerebral stimulant, diaphoretic, diuretic, irritating laxative, respiratory stimulant, and smooth-muscle relaxant. Throughout history it has been used as a remedy for bronchial congestion, constipation (if used occasionally), colds, emphysema, fatigue, headache, jet lag, lethargy, migraines, narcotic poisoning, paralysis, snakebite, and obesity. But few of us can claim to be using coffee medicinally today as we make a beeline for the office coffeemaker.

Coffee is a stimulating, warming, powerful, and addicting substance. In moderation it can help fatigue and promote mental alertness. Caffeine blocks adenosine, a nerve chemical, which tends to make us feel tired. By blocking it, we counter the body's natural rhythms and ignore our impulse to rest. Regular coffee consumption can contribute to an unbalanced emotional state, causing anxiety, panic, stress, nervousness, lack of focus, and insomnia.

Coffee elevates blood sugar levels and stimulates epinephrine production, causing a fight-or-flight response. Eventually our adrenal glands' natural ability to rise to the occasion on their own is diminished.

Coffee increases the heart rate and blood pressure. It can trigger arrthymia and aggravate high blood pressure, acid indigestion, diarrhea, ulcers, and irritable bowel syndrome. It functions as an irritant laxative and can make users dependent on it in order to move their bowels. It also irritates the prostate gland and bladder. Coffee even depletes the body's absorption of nutrients. It inhibits iron and zinc assimilation and, due to its diuretic effect, causes the body to lose valuable water-soluble nutrients such as B-complex vitamins, calcium, and potassium.

Coffee can be particularly disruptive to a woman's reproductive cycle. Women who are prone to breast cysts should avoid coffee altogether, because it can aggravate the condition. It should not be used during pregnancy or while nursing. Research at Johns Hopkins University suggests that women who consume more than three cups of coffee daily decrease their chances of conception by 25 percent. Coffee can also increase the risk of miscarriage, and excessive consumption has been associated with birth defects.

Even decaffeinated coffee is not completely free of caffeine. In addition, it contains the residue of chemicals that can be a health risk, including methylene chloride, which causes toxicity in the liver and cancer in laboratory animals. Water-processed and Swiss-processed decaffeinated coffees are considered safer than the chemically decaffeinated product.

Coffee also often contains residues of dangerous agricultural chemicals. One hundred seventy pesticides are commonly used on coffee plants. Of these, seventy-six are prohibited in the United States because they are dangerous to human health (not only for the coffee imbiber, but for the workers on the coffee plantations as well). So if you do enjoy an occasional cup, buy organic.

To keep your coffee consumption in check without giving it up entirely, try taking a week off from the beverage every once in a while once you have overcome your daily need for caffeine. Some people can enjoy an occasional cup of coffee without becoming dependent on it; others can manage to drink a cup a day. Many people are caffeine sensitive, however, and even low doses can cause nervousness and insomnia. When clients tell me that they only drink a couple of cups of coffee a day, I always ask, "How big are the cups?" When they approximate the size of a ten-inch mug—what most of us are using for a "cup" these days—I make them aware that each of those cups is equal to at least two cups of coffee; they're really drinking about six cups a day.

If you're going to indulge in the occasional cup of coffee, you would do well to drink it mindfully and enjoy it thoroughly. Grind the beans fresh yourself, because coffee can become rancid easily. Set aside the time to sit quietly and do nothing else: savor the aroma and drink it with focus. This is much wiser than hastily gulping a mug while you fight traffic on your way to work.

Tea

Nothing is quite as comforting as a warm cup of tea on a cold day, especially when shared with a friend. New research indicates that tea contains numerous beneficial constituents and suggests that enjoying a few cups a day may actually provide significant health benefits, especially if you choose green tea. But like coffee, tea contains a significant amount of caffeine (green tea contains less than black), which isn't healthy if taken in large amounts. Fewer people in the United States are addicted to tea than to coffee, but tea can be addictive nevertheless. If you brew it strong and drink numerous cups daily, you may be dependent on the caffeine it provides to power you through your day. You can test your dependency by skipping your daily dose (remember to skip the cola, chocolate, and coffee, too!). If you feel fine, then you're in control of your caffeine intake. If you experience withdrawal symptoms, you need to find ways to cut back.

Tea *(Camellia sinensis)* is a member of the Theaceae family. The leaf buds and young leaves are the parts generally used. Processing is what creates the wide variety of flavors found among green and black teas. To make green tea, the leaves and buds are collected, allowed to wilt, then steamed or heated over an open fire. When dried, they retain their green color and are higher in beneficial tannins than black tea leaves. To make black tea, the leaves and buds are twisted, then wilted and fermented, turning the green leaves dark brown. The leaves are then rolled, dried quickly, and sifted into different grades. Kukicha is made from the twigs of the tea plant. Bancha comes from the twigs and older leaves. Oolong tea is partially fermented.

> Legend says that in 2737 B.C., some tea leaves accidentally blew into Emperor Shen-nung's cup of boiling water, thus making the first cup of tea.

Tea has a long and venerable history. It has been used as a stimulating beverage for more than three thousand years in China and Japan. In the early days of seafaring, when scurvy was the bane of sailors around the world, Chinese sailors found themselves relatively immune because they were great drinkers of tea, which contains

Eastern Perspectives on Tea

In traditional Chinese medicine tea is considered energetically bittersweet and drying. Green tea and oolong are cooling, while black tea is warming. Those with a cold constitution will benefit from adding warming spices such as cinnamon or ginger to their tea. Tea is often recommended to enhance digestion, brighten the eyes, open the acupuncture meridians, rejuvenate the spirit, reduce flatulence, and clear the voice. Like coffee, however, in the long term tea can cause depletion of chi.

plenty of vitamin C. Tea also improves digestion, invigorates the mind, and illuminates the spirit—the Japanese often refer to someone who lacks vitality by saying, "He has no tea in him."

Research into tea's benefits is just beginning, but the early results look promising. Both green and black teas are antioxidants, but green tea's healthful properties appear to be far greater. Several recent studies suggest that people who drink green tea regularly may reduce their risk of colorectal, stomach, lung, bladder, esophageal, and pancreatic cancers. Green tea may also protect against skin cancer. According to Japanese research, epigallocatechin, one of the tannins in green tea, protects against cell mutation and possibly cancer. Canadian studies have indicated that the anticancer properties of tea stem from tea's inhibition of nitrosamines, a group of powerful carcinogens. Unfortunately, decaffeinated green tea does not seem to offer the same health benefits, and adding milk to your tea negates these beneficial antioxidant properties as well.

Tea has solventlike properties that break down fats, and when consumed after meals rich in fats, it reduces the risk of arterial disease. Tea also contains theophylline, a close relative of the theobromine found in cocoa. Theophylline stimulates the heart and dilates the airways; it can help improve breathing in those suffering from congestion such as asthma. Tea may also help protect the teeth, although it does stain them if used frequently. Green and black tea prevent dental decay by inhibiting the growth of *Streptococcus mutans,* the bacteria responsible for plaque formation. Tea also contains fluorine, which may help prevent cavities and gum disease.

Tea is also a traditional remedy for allergies, arteriosclerosis, depression, diarrhea, digestive tract infections, dysentery, fatigue, hangovers, hepatitis, high cholesterol, migraines, and scurvy.

While tea may indeed confer some health benefits if used in moderation, addiction to tea isn't healthy. Tea contains much less caffeine than coffee, but the warnings about caffeine's overuse apply equally to the overuse of tea. Pregnant or lactating women should avoid caffeine, as should those with high blood pressure. Like coffee, tea can prevent a migraine when taken at the first sign of one—especially in those who are not regular imbibers—but it can also trigger migraines in those who are hypersensitive. Excessive amounts of tea weaken the kidneys and stomach and can cause constipation or even ulcers. Tea's tannic acid can be mildly irritating to the mucosa of the gastrointestinal tract and can reduce the absorption of the minerals zinc and manganese.

Making the Leap

When you're giving up caffeine, doing so gradually can help prevent withdrawal symptoms such as headaches, lethargy, nausea, vomiting, depression, and irritability. If you stop abruptly, withdrawal symptoms will begin twelve to eighteen hours after the last cup. Start by cutting down gradually—drink one cup less a day—over the course of a week. If you're a coffee drinker, you might then try switching to black tea, which has less caffeine, as you reduce your overall amount of daily caffeine consumption. If you drink black tea, try green tea instead. You might also try a tea made from rooibos *(Aspalathus linearis)* or blackberry *(Rubus fruticosus)* leaf, both of which have a flavor similar to black tea without the caffeine.

> **What Is Rooibos?**
> Native to the mountains of South Africa, rooibos, also known as red bush tea, is just being discovered in North America and Japan. New studies on this ancient plant suggest that it has remarkable healing properties as an antioxidant and adaptogen. It relieves insomnia, anxiety, mild depression, and gastrointestinal distress. The leaves are rich in iron, potassium, calcium, copper, zinc, magnesium, fluoride, and sodium.
>
> To brew a cup of rooibos tea, bring 1 cup of water to a boil. Pour over 1 heaping teaspoon of rooibos leaves. Cover and let steep 10 minutes, then strain and drink.

There also are many excellent coffee substitutes that contain ingredients such as roasted dandelion root, chicory, acorns, and roasted barley. Beverages made from these roots, nuts, and grains have a rich, earthy flavor that will diminish your cravings for coffee.

⸙ Dandelion and Chicory Coffees ⸙

To make dandelion or chicory coffee, you need to roast the roots. Dig up the roots and wash them well, scrubbing off the dirt with a vegetable brush. Slice the roots lengthwise and allow them to dry in a warm, dry location. Once they're dry, roast them in a low oven (about 200 degrees) for about 4 hours, or until brown and crisp. Cool completely, then store in a sealed glass container in a cool, dark location.

To brew a cup of "coffee," use 1 heaping teaspoon of dried roots per cup of water. Either simmer the roots in the water for 10 minutes or, for a drip machine, place them in the paper-lined basket, just as you would ground coffee beans.

⸙ Warming Winter Tea ⸙

This tea can be a good noncaffeinated substitute for coffee.

4 cups springwater
2 teaspoons roasted dandelion roots (see
    instructions for roasting above), crushed
½ teaspoon cinnamon bark, crushed
½ teaspoon dried gingerroot, crushed
½ teaspoon decorticated cardamom pods, crushed
½ teaspoon star anise, crushed
Milk (optional)
Honey (optional)

Bring the water to a boil and then remove from heat. Add the herbs, cover, and let steep 15 minutes. Add milk and honey if desired.

Yerba maté is another good substitute for coffee. It contains mateine, a cousin of caffeine that doesn't have many of caffeine's adverse effects. Yerba maté is a pleasant stimulant that is nonaddictive, is rich in nutrients, and doesn't contribute to anxiety or insomnia. Green tea is another option; it contains much less caffeine and offers other important health benefits. Researchers report that green tea is a powerful antioxidant, more effective than vitamins C or E. Drinking green tea regularly may help prevent cancer, cardiovascular disease, and liver disorders. It will give you a gentle lift with healthier fringe benefits!

Herbal Therapy

Other herbs to use for energy and a clear mind include the following:

- **Ginseng** helps the body adapt to stress. It nourishes the adrenal glands and promotes mental and physical alertness.
- **Ginkgo** improves circulation, thus boosting mental alertness.
- **Nettle** helps repair intestines harmed by excess coffee consumption.

Nutrition Therapy

One of the best ways to reduce stress in your life is to reduce your intake of stimulants such as coffee and tea. The important question to ask yourself is, *Why am I using stimulants?* If you have a problem waking up in the morning, try going to sleep an hour earlier at night and have an energizing breakfast—not a jelly doughnut. Starting your day with a warm mug of miso broth (see the following recipe) is a body-friendly way to energize yourself. And turn to the section Overcoming Fatigue and Increasing Energy (see page 212) and pay attention. Exercising first thing in the morning stimulates endorphin production and can help you to feel more alive and alert. If your energy tends to flag later in the day, take along high-protein snacks to munch on, such as sunflower and pumpkin seeds or roasted nuts. Try some nourishing tonics such as green barley juice or ginseng. Deep-breathing exercises can also be a chemical-free way to energize mental alertness.

Is coffee your thing because you would be constipated without it? Add a handful of flaxseeds to your daily diet and things should come out just fine. You can also try drinking a glass of hot or room-temperature water with a squeeze of lemon.

♪ Morning Miso ♭

Begin your morning by recharging your long-term energy reserves with a warming cup of miso broth. Just stir 1 teaspoon of miso into 1 cup of hot water. You can find miso in your local health foods store. The yellow and white varieties tend to be lower in sodium.

Aromatherapy

Aromatherapy is a wonderful way to perk yourself up. In the morning try a dry-brush skin massage (see the full instructions in chapter 9), then shower with peppermint soap and end with a quick cold-water rinse. That will get you going!

You can also use inhalations of essential oils that will support and energize you while you're giving up caffeine.

- **For coffee,** try cardamom, cinnamon, juniper, sandalwood, and vanilla.
- **For tea,** try geranium, lemon, and peppermint.

Do you get tired at work? Take some stretching breaks or short walks and spritz yourself with some uplifting aromatherapy sprays made from diluted peppermint, lavender, or rosemary essential oils. Just mix 20 drops of essential oil with 1 tablespoon of vinegar and 8 ounces of water. Shake well and spritz your face and neck (keeping eyes and mouth closed!) whenever you start to drag.

You can also keep a bottle of essential oil at your desk for an emergency pick-me-up. Put a drop on a handkerchief or tissue and inhale deeply.

5

You Can't Eat Your Way to Happiness

Overcoming Food Addictions

Food addiction can cause as much suffering and have as many negative health consequences as any other addiction. Although America is the land of plenty—or perhaps because of it—it's also the homeland of a wide range of eating disorders. Because food is necessary, available, and legal, not many people consider it a source of addiction. But for some people, certain foods can be as addictive as alcohol and cocaine.

Food addictions have many physical side effects, including poor concentration, fatigue, diarrhea, constipation, bloating, skin disorders, and fluid retention. They also have powerful emotional and psychological side effects, including anxiety, depression, loss of self-esteem, and poor self-confidence.

The Sugar Connection

Sugar dependencies lie at the root of many addictions, especially food addictions. When blood sugar levels are low, you can experience nervous tension, irritability, and depression. Eating—especially eating something with simple sugars in it—quickly elevates blood sugar levels and makes you feel better. Many alcoholics and other addicts find that they become addicted to sweets after getting sober. In these cases, they've simply substituted one form of sugar addiction for another. For many others, refined carbohydrates such as white flour trigger addiction. And as you've seen in chapter 3, the sugar dependency cycle has terrible effects on the body.

Food Allergies and Sensitivities

Very often we crave the foods we're allergic to. If you consume a food that you're allergic or sensitive to, you may initially experience an increase in metabolism, causing an energy rush. As this feeling wears off and you return to normal, you feel a decrease in energy, which leads to a craving for the food that stimulated the high. Common allergens include wheat, dairy products, eggs, corn, sugar, yeast, citrus, peanuts, chocolate, coffee, soy, potatoes, tomatoes, and shellfish.

If you suspect that you're allergic to a particular food, have an allergy test done. There's also a simple way to test for a food allergy at home. Check your pulse on an empty stomach; count the number of pulses you feel for six seconds, then multiply that number by ten to determine your pulse per minute. Thirty to sixty minutes after a meal, check your pulse again. If it's faster than it was on an empty stomach, this may be a signal that you're having a reaction to a food you consumed.

Are You a Food Addict?

The most common characteristic of food addicts is that they eat compulsively with no regard for the consequences. They are persistently preoccupied with buying, preparing, and eating food. Sneaking or stealing food, hiding food, hiding signs of eating food—such as discarding empty wrappers in the bottom of the wastebasket—can all be indicators of food addiction. Food addicts may also feel uneasy when food is not available, gobble food quickly with little chewing, obsess about weight, and consistently continue to eat after others have stopped.

As with any other addiction, a food addiction can be caused by a biochemical imbalance. A food addict may be unable to quit after one bite of a trigger or "binge" food, just as an alcoholic may be unable to stop drinking after just one sip. The food addict may develop a tolerance so that larger and larger amounts of a food are required to satisfy cravings. When the food supply is cut off, withdrawal symptoms can occur, including chills, dizziness, nausea, headaches, lethargy, and inability to concentrate. Similar to drug and alcohol withdrawal, a person not getting his or her food "fix" may experience flulike symptoms, even to the point of being bedridden.

In many cases people who binge on food use laxatives, diuretics, and self-induced vomiting to purge their bodies of the huge quantities they have eaten. Not only are these techniques ineffective—most bingeing is done with refined carbohydrates, which are very quickly absorbed—but they can have devastating effects upon the body over the long term.

> **Bulimia**
>
> *Bulimia* derives from the Greek for "ox hunger." Common among food addicts, bulimia is a repeated cycle of eating excessively, or bingeing, and then purging, either by vomiting or through the abuse of laxatives. It may be aggravated by a lack of or inactivity of the hormonelike substance cholecystokinin (CCK), which signals the brain that the stomach is full. Bulimia has devastating effects on the body and can be fatal. It's classified as a psychiatric disorder.

The Chemistry of Binge Eating

Binge eating creates a chemical dependency on the feel-good neurotransmitters that the behavior produces, namely serotonin and endorphins.

Most people with food addictions overeat sugars and refined carbohydrates. These stimulate the brain to release serotonin, a calming neurotransmitter that helps ease feelings of stress and is supposed to reduce cravings for more carbohydrates. However, when you're hooked on that feeling of serenity and well-being, your body can override the message, *You don't need anymore carbohydrates.*

Binge eating also causes a release of endorphins, which reduce tension and elevate mood. Both anorexics and bulimics tend to have abnormally low endorphin levels. Excessive dieting or starving, binge-ing, purging, and overexercising all elevate endorphin levels, which can make it difficult for people with eating disorders to change.

Behavior Therapy

When you experience a food craving, remind yourself that most crav-ings pass in just a few minutes. Take a few deep, slow breaths. Relax.

Don't allow food to be the greatest source of comfort and pleasure in your life. Consider the sensual delights of taking a warm bubble bath, getting a massage, reading a great novel, or walking in a beauti-ful environment—be it nature or an art museum. Practice prayer, meditation, guided visualization, and yoga to enhance serenity and stability in your life.

Exercise is essential to giving up a food addiction; like binge eat-ing, exercise stimulates endorphin release—but much more safely! It also warms the body, improves digestion, and inhibits the spleen from turning phlegm to fat. It can improve posture, energy levels, circula-tion, and elimination and help the body make better use of oxygen. However, remember that excessive exercise can have the opposite effect, causing exhaustion and depletion.

Keep a food journal. Record in it what you eat and drink—every last bite or sip—for a week to gain insight about what your diet really looks like.

Keep a weekly shopping list and stick with it. Avoid the aisles in the grocery store that are filled with food banished from your diet. When at restaurants, order first so you don't get swayed by others' choices.

Eat only when you're hungry!

Too often mealtime is simply a rushed continuation of the stress in our daily lives. Instead, make it a time to sit back, relax, and enjoy being with yourself and your family. Make eating a ritual, not some-thing that must be rushed through right away. Serve food on beauti-ful plates, rather than eating out of containers. Serve small portions to the table rather than having country-style help-yourself platters. Sit down, relax, look at your food, and say a blessing or take a few deep breaths to calm and center yourself.

On the average it takes the brain twenty minutes to realize that the stomach is satisfied. So slow down and enjoy what you eat. Put your fork down between bites. Be mindful of the experience. Don't read or watch TV while you're eating. When you feel 70 percent full, stop eating.

Snacks are a necessary part of the day, especially if you're eating small meals. But remember—eat only if you're hungry! Avoid carbohydrate snacks such as pretzels and crackers; instead focus on protein- and calcium-rich snacks such as nuts and yogurt. Don't snack in the evening after dinner. Instead, immediately after eating, brush and floss your teeth to discourage anymore food consumption.

Family and professional support as well as nutritional therapy can help a person to find the road back to health. Though most addicts need to practice total abstinence when giving up an addiction to stay clean, food addicts need to find balance. Set goals for yourself, and use this as an opportunity to live a healthier lifestyle that can add years and joy to your life.

Nutritional Therapy

To overcome a food addiction, you must totally abstain from whatever foods make you feel like bingeing. In most cases this means all forms of refined carbohydrates, including bread, pasta, crackers, cake, pizza, bagels, muffins, croissants, and so on, and anything with sugar in it. Read ingredients lists. You'll be surprised to see how many prepackaged foods contain outrageous amounts of sugar. And, of course, you must abstain from any foods that you think you are allergic or sensitive to.

Instead, satisfy your food cravings with protein-rich foods such as legumes, tofu, tempeh, eggs, fish, and lean poultry. Also include some naturally sweet foods such as baked winter squash, carrots, and millet.

Avoid alcohol due to its high sugar and grain content. Eliminate caffeine, which can aggravate feelings of anxiety or depression and increase the desire to binge eat.

Make sea vegetables, such as kelp, dulse, and hiziki, a part of your diet. These are a good source of nutritive minerals and also improve thyroid function, which can pep up a sluggish metabolism. Sea vegetables are also available in tablet or capsule form. Other foods that are satisfying and cleansing in nature include miso soup, barley, steamed vegetables, daikon radish, and celery.

Consuming a heaping teaspoon of psyllium husk stirred into water or a handful of freshly ground flaxseeds daily will cause you to feel full and help lubricate the bowels, promoting good elimination. However, when using these two food supplements, it's imperative to consume plenty of fluids; otherwise they could cause constipation.

If you're craving for something sweet, your body may be trying to tell you that you need more protein. Try snacking on a handful of nuts or pumpkin or sunflower seeds. Or eat something naturally sweet, such as an apple. Take a dose of herbal bitters to dispel the craving.

If you're craving something salty, your body may be trying to tell you that you need more minerals, such as those found in sea vegetables. Try eating some brown rice rolled up in seaweed.

If you're craving fats, you could be lacking in essential fatty acids (EFAs) or protein. Take a tablespoon daily of flaxseed or hempseed oil, both good sources of EFAs. Eat more eggs, fish, lean poultry, and legumes, which are good sources of protein.

Herbal Therapy

The following herbs can help you kick a food addiction:

- **Alfalfa** is highly nutritive, providing a wealth of vitamins and minerals that satisfy the body's needs. It also contains enzymes that aid in digestion.
- **Amla** is rich in nutrients, especially vitamin C. It's mildly laxative; in Ayurvedic medicine it's said to help you feel lighter and happier.
- **Burdock** improves the function of many of the organs of elimination, including the kidneys, liver, and bowel. It aids in fat metabolism and is slightly diuretic.
- **Cardamom** improves circulation to the digestive system and enhances the body's ability to digest grains and dairy products.

- **Cayenne** is considered a thermogenic herb, meaning that it revs up metabolism and thus can aid in weight loss. It improves fat metabolism and stimulates the brain to release endorphins.
- **Cinnamon** is naturally sweet and can curb the desire for other sugars. It's warming and improves circulation.
- **Codonopsis** is also naturally sweet and can curb the desire for other sugars. It's a tonic for the spleen and stomach, can help you acclimate to stress, and is highly nutritive.
- **Cola nut** contains caffeine and theobromine, which are stimulants. In West Africa chewing on cola nuts is a traditional way to allay hunger and relieve mental exhaustion.
- **Dandelion root** improves liver function and thus the metabolism of fats. The leaf is a natural diuretic and is rich in trace minerals, especially potassium.
- **Ephedra** can curb appetite and enhance energy. Ephedra should not be used by everyone nor for extended periods of time, however; see the precautions listed in chapter 2.
- **Fennel seed** is a natural appetite suppressant.
- **Garcinia** inhibits the conversion of excess calories into fat. It also raises blood sugar levels, curbing the desire for sweets.
- **Gentian** is a bitter tonic that aids in the metabolism of fats and proteins. It also improves assimilation of iron and vitamin B12.
- **Ginger** improves circulation to all parts of the body. It aids digestion and is energizing.
- **Green tea** is a diuretic; it contains caffeine and is thus a stimulant, but it's more gentle than coffee. It aids in the breakdown of cholesterol and helps keep blood sugar levels on an even keel.
- **Gymnema**, when consumed before eating, blocks the taste and metabolism of sugar, which can quickly help your body kick a sugar dependency.
- **Hawthorn leaves, flowers, and berries** are used in traditional Chinese medicine to enhance weight loss. They help break down fatty deposits, are mildly diuretic, and energize the body.
- **Horsetail** is highly nutritive and mildly diuretic.
- **Nettle** is highly nutritive, diuretic, energizing, and a circulatory stimulant. It's a traditional remedy for cellulite.

- **Parsley** is nutritive and diuretic. It has a high chlorophyll content, which enables the body to make better use of oxygen. It also increases circulation to the digestive tract.
- **St. John's wort** is a natural antidepressant. It calms anxiety and quiets the nerves.
- **Turmeric** aids in fat metabolism, improves elimination, and helps stabilize the body's microflora, thus inhibiting yeast overgrowth, which can contribute to food addictions.
- **Valerian root** is a sedative and nervine. It can help curb overeating caused by stress or anxiety.
- **Yerba maté** functions as an appetite suppressant, an antidepressant, and a mild stimulant. It's also rich in minerals and vitamins.

Supplement Therapy

Sweet cravings can be reduced by taking spirulina capsules daily. They're available at most natural foods stores; just follow the dosage directions on the package. Other supplements to consider are as follows:

SUPPLEMENT	DOSAGE	COMMENTS
GTF chromium	200–1,000 mcg daily	Helps reduce carbohydrate as well as sugar cravings.
Zinc	30–60 mg daily	Low levels of zinc have been associated with both anorexia and bulimia.
Flaxseed or hempseed oil	1–3 tbsps. daily	Rich in essential fatty acids, which can help improve the body's metabolism of fat and reduce fat cravings.
Lecithin granules	1–3 tbsps. daily	Aids in fat metabolism.
L-glutamine	250–1,000 mg daily	Reduces sugar and carbohydrate cravings.

Hydrotherapy

One technique for getting into better touch with your body is the dry-brush skin massage. Before bathing, gently massage your skin with a natural-fiber brush. Brush in circular strokes, starting with your feet, then your legs, then your arms, and finally your torso, always moving toward the heart. Dry brushing is stimulating and energizing, improves circulation, and aids in the elimination of toxins. Afterward, soak in a relaxing herbal bath, such as the one suggested below.

⸱ Slimming Herbal Bath ⸱
A small handful each of dulse, thyme, peppermint, and rosemary
A dark-colored washcloth or sachet bag

Place the herbs in the center of the cloth. Tie the cloth with a hair tie, throw it in the tub, and start running a hot bath. When it's full enough, turn off the faucets and allow the water to cool until it feels comfortable to bathe in. While bathing, enjoy the pleasant fragrance and use the herb-filled cloth to gently scrub your body.

Aromatherapy

Inhalations of various essential oils can quell cravings and improve your self-control.

- **Anise, fennel, and spearmint** essential oils are naturally sweet and dispel unnecessary urges to eat.
- **Grapefruit** essential oil helps those who eat when under pressure.
- **Bergamot** essential oil helps deter food addictions.
- **Bitter orange** essential oil helps deter sweet cravings.

6

Up in Smoke
Beating the Nicotine Fix

The tobacco plant is native to North and South America; indigenous peoples there used its leaves for healing and in spiritual ceremonies. When European explorers first reached the Americas, they were curious to know more about this sacred herb. They learned to grow it, and they carried samples back with them to Europe. Five centuries later we find ourselves in a world inundated with chemical-laden tobacco mixes and plagued by tobacco abuse. More than three million people die every year of cancers stemming from tobacco use. What happened?

A Brief History

When Columbus arrived in the New World in the late fifteenth century, he was given gifts of fruits and "certain dried leaves" by the Arawak tribe, the first Native Americans he met. The gifts seemed prized, and he accepted them. Not knowing what to do with the strange leaves, he later threw them away. Others who followed in his footsteps were not so hasty.

Within the space of a few decades more Spaniards were converted to tobacco than Indians to Christianity. European explorers and colonists touting tobacco's medicinal properties introduced it to Europe. It wasn't long before vast expanses of North American forests were cleared to make way for tobacco growing.

The custom of smoking tobacco rolled in paper began in Spain in the seventeenth century and gradually spread. Before the invention of cigarette-rolling machines in the nineteenth century, tobacco was hand-rolled, snuffed, chewed, or smoked in pipes—and the inconvenience of these methods most likely limited their use. In addition, smoking was not an acceptable social behavior in many circles at the time. In fact, ten states had laws against smoking. By World War I, however, smoking had become an integral part of North American culture. Cigarettes were distributed free to soldiers, and it became customary even for women to smoke. At last count (a 1997 National Health Interview Survey), forty-eight million adults in the United States were regular smokers.

Tobacco's Medicinal Uses

Tobacco wasn't arbitrarily chosen as a sacred herb by Native Americans. Like most plants, tobacco has some medicinal properties. It's an anaphrodisiac, antispasmodic, cardiovascular stimulant, depressant, diaphoretic, emetic, and stimulant. It has been used to soothe anxiety, reduce appetite, combat fatigue, and stimulate mental function. Tobacco juice can be applied topically to kill worms and lice and to treat wounds, swellings, ulcerations, snakebites, and scorpion stings; tobacco smoke blown gently into the ear can soothe an earache. Tobacco "tea" is a potent insecticide, especially against aphids, and is often used in commercial agriculture.

On the whole, however, tobacco is highly toxic. Chewing on tobacco leaf or drinking an infusion of tobacco can lead to vomiting,

Chewing tobacco, pipes, and cigars are as addictive and dangerous as cigarettes. Although most of this chapter will focus on cigarettes, the advice and remedies given are also effective for those wanting to beat addiction to these alternative forms of tobacco.

convulsions, and possible respiratory failure. Nicotine, one of the most notorious alkaloids in tobacco, is a known poison; taken in large enough doses, it can lethally paralyze the breathing muscles. Cigarettes deliver nicotine only in small amounts that the body can quickly break down and get rid of, which is why the nicotine does not kill instantly. These small doses, however, are enough to cause dizziness, sweating, and heart palpitations in those whose bodies haven't built up a tolerance.

The Smoker's High

Cigarettes function as both stimulant and sedative. Tobacco leaves are cured in sugar; when smoked, they raise blood sugar levels. In response to cigarettes, the body produces epinephrine, which helps eliminate the smoke's toxins by speeding up the metabolic process. Circulation increases; blood vessels constrict; the heart starts to beat faster.

Later, as the body rids itself of the nicotine, heart rate and other body functions slow down. The smoker may initially feel relaxed, then later a bit uncomfortable and depressed. Blood sugar levels drop. At this point the smoker will feel anxious to have another smoke.

Smoking and Women

Smoking holds unique risks for women. Women over the age of thirty-five who smoke and use the Pill (oral contraceptives) are in a high-risk group for heart attack, stroke, and blood clots of the legs. They are also more likely to have miscarriages or babies with low birth weight.

Deciding to Quit

If you want to quit smoking, you're not alone. According to a 1995 study by the Centers for Disease Control (CDC), almost 70 percent of smokers in the United States want to quit, and half of them attempt to do so every year. In 1995, 23 percent of the adults in the United States—25 million men and 19.3 million women—were former smokers.

Unfortunately, quitting smoking is a difficult undertaking. The nicotine found in cigarettes, cigars, and chewing tobacco is highly addictive. Teenagers in particular find it very difficult to quit— according to the CDC, 73 percent of teens who have ever smoked daily have tried to quit, but only 14 percent have been successful. In fact, the 1990–92 National Comorbidity Survey estimated that of people aged fifteen through twenty-four, almost 24 percent of those who had ever smoked cigarettes went on to become addicted. This parallels the use-to-dependence conversion rates for cocaine (25 percent) and heroin (20 percent)!

The Dangers of Smoking

Modern cigarette production is a very toxic endeavor: Herbicides and pesticides are used in the tobacco fields, chemicals are added to the tobacco mix to enhance burning, and the rolling papers are processed with heavy-duty bleaches. Cigarette smoke contains many lethal gases, including carbon monoxide, nitrogen, hydrogen cyanide, and sulfur oxides, as well as tar, which is composed of more than four thousand different chemical constituents, including forty-three known carcinogens. Is it any wonder that smoking makes us sick?

In today's society just about everyone is well versed in the dangerous relationship between lung cancer and smoking. However, few people realize that smoking has also been implicated in myriad other cancers and health problems. According to the American Cancer Society's Cancer Prevention Study II, from 1990 through 1994 nearly one in five deaths in the United States were attributable to smoking.

- **Cancer.** Tobacco use accounts for 30 percent, or one in three, of all cancer deaths in the United States. Scientific research has proven that cigarette smoking is a major cause of cancers of the lung, larynx, mouth, pharynx, and esophagus and is a contributing cause in the development of cancers of the bladder, pancreas, cervix, and kidney. Chewing tobacco, cigar and pipe smoking, and tobacco snuff, in particular, are linked to a higher incidence of tongue, mouth, and throat cancer. Melanoma, or cancer of the skin, is more likely to spread through the bodies of smokers than of non-smokers.

The American Cancer Society estimates that smoking decreases a person's life span by about fifteen years.

• **Lung disease.** Cigarette smoking causes several lung diseases that can be just as dangerous as lung cancer. Two of the most common are chronic bronchitis and emphysema.

A person with bronchitis suffers from inflammation in the bronchial tubes and excess mucus in the airways, which often causes him or her to cough frequently and uncontrollably. Chronic bronchitis is a repeating incidence of this illness.

Emphysema is a degenerative disease that slowly destroys a person's ability to breathe. The surface of the lungs is covered in thousands of alveoli. When you breathe in, the alveoli stretch as they transport oxygen from the air to the blood. When you breathe out, the alveoli constrict to force out carbon dioxide. Smoking can cause the walls of these cells to become less elastic and eventually to break down, resulting in larger but fewer sacs. Exhaling becomes difficult, because the damaged alveoli have air trapped inside them and lack the elasticity to force it out in exchange for fresh air. As the damage progresses, each breath becomes more labored.

• **Heart disease.** High blood presssure, high cholesterol, and a sedentary lifestyle are all factors in the incidence of heart disease, but only smoking doubles that risk. In addition, smokers who have had a heart attack are more likely than nonsmokers to have another attack. Smoking a pack of cigarettes a day—that's twenty cigarettes—can make you three times more likely to have a heart attack and five times more likely to suffer a stroke than nonsmokers. Women who smoke and take birth control pills are at even greater risk.

• **Poor nutrition.** Smoking one cigarette destroys about twenty-five milligrams of vitamin C. Smokers almost always have less vitamin C in their bodies than do nonsmokers. The longer you've smoked, the less vitamin C you have in your system. Without vitamin C, your body's cells are more likely to suffer from free-radical damage—and free radicals are a by-product of cigarette smoke. A vitamin C deficiency can contribute to hardening of the arteries, which is common in smokers. In addition, nicotine has been found to stimulate digestive secretions and shorten bowel transit time, thus decreasing the nutrients available to the body.

- **Decreased immune system function.** Of all the addictive substances, tobacco is one of the most damaging to the immune system. Tobacco stuns the cilia, the small hairs that act as natural filters in the air passages and keep foreign particles out of the lungs. When these cilia become paralyzed, foreign particles have free access to the lungs, increasing the risk of infection. Smoking also causes more mucus to be produced, creating a breeding ground for bacteria and making you more prone to respiratory infection such as emphysema and bronchitis. In addition, smoking impairs immune activity by increasing suppressor T cells and decreasing helper T cells. Smokers in general have higher levels of white blood cells, which increase in the presence of infection and inflammation in the body.

- **Poor reproductive health.** Smoking can cause men to have a lower sperm count, more abnormal sperm, and sperm with less motility. Because smoking causes constriction of peripheral blood vessels, it can also impair blood flow to the penis and make a full erection unlikely.

In a study conducted by the Oxford Family Planning Association, of four thousand women, those who smoked more than sixteen cigarettes daily were twice as likely not to conceive as nonsmokers. Pregnant women who smoke share with their unborn child all of the side effects of smoking: nicotine enters the placenta and amniotic fluid, and the fetus's blood vessels become constricted, lowering fetal blood supply and decreasing the amount of oxygen and nutrients available to the baby.

Pregnant women who smoke have more miscarriages and stillbirths and usually give birth to smaller babies. After birth, smoking is still a risk. Nicotine enters the breast milk and can decrease the amount produced in nursing mothers. Babies

**Eastern Perspectives
on Tobacco**

In traditional Chinese medicine tobacco is considered energetically hot. It heats the body, particularly the lungs. Tobacco is bitter and dry and is harmful to the chi and yin (fluids) of the lungs. In the short term, smoking tobacco can be relaxing, because the heat of the inhaled smoke disperses stagnant chi from the lungs. Tar and nicotine buildup in the lungs causes chi stagnation, however, and smoking soon becomes a cycle of chi release and stagnation. In addition, when the lungs are hot and dry, as from smoking, they become easy targets for cancer.

whose mothers smoke are at higher risk for asthma, colds, ear infections, and other respiratory diseases as well as sudden infant death syndrome (SIDS).

• **Premature aging.** Nicotine decreases circulation to both the organs and the skin, causing smokers to age more quickly on the inside and the outside. Smoking creates skin that's dry, wrinkled, leathery, and grayish yellow in tone—not a pretty picture! Women who smoke reach menopause at an earlier age, though the reason is not certain; many scientists believe that smoking is related to reduced estrogen levels, which may also be why women smokers are at a higher risk for osteoporosis.

• **Decreased circulation.** Because nicotine decreases circulation, which drastically reduces blood flow to the extremities, smokers tend to have cold hands and feet. Smoking is also a contributing factor in Buerger's disease, a circulatory disease characterized by blood clots and severe pain, usually in the legs.

• **Digestive disorders.** Smokers experience more digestive disorders, including heartburn, diverticulosis, and indigestion, than nonsmokers. Smoking can contribute to the development of peptic ulcers, and in general ulcers take longer to heal in smokers than in nonsmokers.

• **Diminished eyesight.** Smoke is an eye irritant and can damage the eyes' internal structure. In 1974 a study conducted by the Smoking Research Center of San Diego and the U.S. Department of Health, Education, and Welfare demonstrated that both nicotine and carbon monoxide decreased oxygen supply to the eyes, diminishing eyesight and creating tunnel vision. Smoking can also be a factor in photophobia, or light sensitivity. Smokers also have a higher risk of cataracts than nonsmokers.

- **Gum disease.** In addition to causing cancer of the mouth, tobacco smoke is associated with increased susceptibility to tooth loss and periodontal disease.
- **Alzheimer's disease.** Nicotine has a strong effect on the central nervous system. Initially, smoking causes enhanced learning, memory, and alertness. However, studies have shown that those who smoke more than a pack a day are more likely to develop Alzheimer's disease than nonsmokers.
- **Depression.** Nicotine stimulates a reduction in serotonin levels, which can be a factor in depression. In addition, smokers tend to suffer from insomnia more often than nonsmokers, which can also contribute to depression.

Secondhand Smoke

If you can't quit for yourself, quit for your family and friends. Secondhand smoke is a potent human carcinogen. According to the American Cancer Society, almost forty thousand people die every year from heart disease as a result of breathing secondhand smoke. Exposure to secondhand smoke causes 150,000 to 300,000 respiratory infections (such as pneumonia and bronchitis) every year in children younger than eighteen months. And secondhand smoke can greatly increase a child's risk for asthma, the incidence of asthma attacks, and the severity of those attacks.

Quitting Changes You—For the Better!

To quit smoking, you must break yourself of two dependencies: physically, you must make your body go through the nicotine withdrawal symptoms; psychologically, you must give up the habit of smoking. Withdrawal symptoms can include depression, irritability, frustration, restlessness, insomnia, difficulty concentrating, headaches, lethargy, and increased appetite. They can last from a few days to several weeks. Is quitting worth all this? You bet.

After twenty minutes without a cigarette, heart rate and blood pressure fall to normal levels. After eight hours, carbon monoxide levels

> **If You Must Smoke**
>
> If you are going to continue to smoke, select brands that are chemical-free. Natural tobaccos pose somewhat less of a cancer and heart disease risk. Don't bother with "light" cigarettes—according to a 1997 study by the Massachusetts Department of Public Health, there are no significant differences in the total nicotine content of full-flavor and light cigarettes.

drop to normal. After only twenty-four hours, the risk of heart attack decreases. Forty-eight hours after the last smoke, the senses of smell and taste are already improved. After seventy-two hours of not smoking, breathing becomes easier. After two weeks, lung function and circulation improve. Within the first smoke-free year, coughing, sinus congestion, shortness of breath, and risk of coronary heart disease decrease. In addition, the natural cilia regrow, reducing the risk of lung infection. After five years, the risk of lung cancer drops, and it continues to drop commensurate with the number of smoke-free years that follow.

Behavior Therapy

Once you've made the decision to quit smoking, think about the situations in which you smoke. Is it when you're bored or stressed, in certain social situations, or with certain beverages? For example, some people smoke when they're under pressure; others smoke at social gatherings, after dinner, or when they're out with their friends. Avoid those situations, or substitute a better habit—going for a walk, chewing sugar-free gum, drinking mineral water—for the smoking habit.

Set a smoke-free target date, whether that be a week or a month into the future. Give yourself an allottment of cigarettes to smoke each day and, as you approach the target date, start cutting back on that number.

There are several tactics you can use to help yourself cut back and, eventually, quit:

- When you feel a craving for a cigarette, *delay*. Wait five extra minutes before lighting up. As you approach your target date, make yourself wait longer and longer.
- Pick certain hours of the day when you won't smoke; for example,

Once you've quit, you may find yourself in situations where you're surrounded by smokers. If so, try setting out bowls of apple cider vinegar and burning beeswax candles to absorb some of the smoke.

from 6 A.M. to 9 A.M. and from 6 P.M. to 9 P.M. As you approach your target date, keep extending these smoke-free time periods.

- Smoke only half of each cigarette.
- Keep switching brands. Don't buy your favorite brand.
- Avoid deeply inhaling the first few puffs of each cigarette.
- If you've made it through a smoke-free time period, don't use a cigarette as your reward. Think of something else you can use, such as dropping money into a jar reserved for funds to buy something nice for yourself.
- Before lighting up, ask yourself, *Am I smoking because I really want to, or am I smoking out of habit?*
- When you're smoking, hold each inhalation of smoke in your mouth for thirty seconds while focusing on the negative aspects of smoking. This technique has proven to be successful in many stop-smoking clinics.
- Find a substitute habit for those times when you were accustomed to smoking. For example, if you used to smoke after the dinner meal, go for a walk instead, or use a minty mouthwash or sugar-free mint after a meal to please your mouth and taste buds.
- Take a couple of brisk walks daily in fresh air to get more oxygen into your lungs. Exercise helps reduce stress and increase energy.
- Try rolling your own cigarettes using a mixture of tobacco and other herbs (see page 147 for suggestions). Gradually reduce the amount of tobacco and increase the amount of herbs. Then gradually reduce the number of times you smoke until you're not smoking at all.
- Practice your breathwork. Whenever you feel the desire to smoke, instead focus on deep diaphragmatic breathing. Inhale deeply and slowly, letting your abdomen fill up and expand. Exhale deeply and slowly, feeling your abdomen sinking in. By breathing more deeply and slowly, you feed your body more oxygen. See page 22 in chapter 2 for more deep-breathing exercises.

- If you've been using chewing tobacco, substitute herbal chew formulas, which are available in flavors such as cinnamon, licorice, mint, and wintergreen in many natural foods stores.

Once you've reached your smoke-free target date, don't tell yourself and others that "I'm trying to quit"; instead say, "I quit." Get rid of your smoking paraphernalia. Make an appointment to get your teeth cleaned.

Nutritional Therapy

Tobacco addiction, like most addictions, has roots in low blood sugar. Tobacco intake causes the liver to release more glycogen, which temporarily elevates blood sugar levels. To stabilize blood sugar levels, eat small frequent meals that contain adequate protein from sources such as legumes, fish, poultry, and whole grains such as brown rice, millet, corn, and buckwheat.

Other good foods to help you quit the tobacco habit include:

- **Oats.** Eat oats regularly; they can curb the desire for nicotine.
- **Yogurt** helps calm the nerves.
- **Sunflower seeds.** Eating sunflower seeds, especially the ones that have to be shelled, is nourishing, satisfying, and keeps the hands busy.
- **Ginger.** Eat pieces of crystallized ginger to open the lungs (but rinse off the sugar first).
- **Alkalinizing foods.** A body that is more acidic is more likely to crave cigarettes. Eat alkalinizing foods such as apples, almonds, beet greens, berries, carrots, celery, dandelion greens, figs, lima beans, onions, peas, raisins, and spinach to curb this desire.
- **High-chlorophyll vegetables.** Be sure to include lots of high-chlorophyll vegetables such as collards and kale, which help the body better utilize oxygen.
- **Food rich in beta-carotene** such as carrots and winter squash have been found to help decrease the possibility of lung cancer.
- **High-sulfur foods.** Like foods rich in beta-carotene, high-sulfur

vegetables such as broccoli and cabbage have been found to
help decrease the possibility of lung cancer.

- **High-fiber foods.** Quitting smoking causes a decrease in digestive stimulation, so you're more likely to be constipated. High-
  fiber foods such as oat bran, flaxseeds, carrots, celery, and sweet
  potatoes will help prevent constipation. In addition, be sure to
  drink plenty of water.
- **Fresh vegetable juice.** Drinking fresh vegetable juice will help
  detoxify the body. Celery, beet, wheat grass, and carrot juice are
  helpful; they encourage cleansing of the body and provide valuable antioxidants. Because they're sweet, juices should be diluted
  by half with springwater.

Linus Pauling conducted a study in England in which smokers,
when craving a cigarette, simply took an orange, made a hole in it, and
sucked out the juice. Within three weeks participants showed a 79 percent overall decrease in cigarette consumption, and 20 percent had quit
altogether. The technique may work for two reasons. First, oranges are
high in vitamin C, which can reduce cravings and help detoxify the
body. Second, oranges have natural sugars, and getting that sugar by
sucking an implement about the same size and shape as a cigarette may
help the body break its psychological dependency on cigarettes.

Oral-Manual Therapy

Aside from breaking the nicotine addiction, one of the hardest
aspects of quitting smoking is giving up regular hand-to-mouth
activity, or what many call the oral fixation. Once you've quit smoking, you may find yourself chewing on toothpicks, enjoying lollipops,
and searching for something to occupy your now-fidgety hands.

Don't let yourself substitute food for cigarettes. Weight gain is one
of the most common side effects of quitting smoking. Here are some
better methods to help satisfy the oral-manual fixation:

- Chew on a licorice root, birch tree stick, or other safe, pleasant-
  tasting natural object.

- Mock-smoke a cinnamon stick.
- Sip water through a straw.
- Take up a craft or activity that keeps your hands occupied. Use Chinese hand balls, play with a yo-yo, knit, build a paper clip chain, learn oragami—whatever it takes to keep yourself smoke-free.

Herbs for Tobacco Addiction

There are several herbal preparations—available in natural foods stores in the form of teas, extracts, or capsules—designed to help people give up smoking. In addition, you can fine-tune your own herbal regimen by trying some of the following time-tested stop-smoking aids:

- **Ashwagandha, asparagus root, and marsh mallow root** are lung tonics that nourish, tone, and support lung function.
- **Cloves** stimulate lung circulation, contain valuable antioxidants, and give your mouth a fresh, clean flavor. To help overcome the oral-manual habit as well as the physical dependency, suck on a whole clove.
- **Garlic** can be taken during the cutting-back period to help open the lungs.
- **Ginger** helps increase circulation to the lungs, which in turn helps move toxins and reduces inflammation in lung tissue. You can take ginger supplements as described in chapter 2, or you can chew on fresh ginger slices or pieces of candied ginger (wash off the sugar first so that you don't feed a sugar dependency).
- **Ginseng** helps the body better utilize oxygen and aids in keeping blood sugar levels steady.
- **Juniper berry** can help open and detoxify the lungs. Try chewing on five berries a day.
- **Lobelia** contains the alkaloid lobeline, which helps satisfy the body's craving for nicotine.
- **Magnolia** is drying the the throat, which can make smoking unpleasant, and it has cleansing and diaphoretic properties.
- **Marjoram** is also drying to the throat, and it increases circula-

tion to the lungs, which can help move the toxins that have collected there.

- **Mullein** is an expectorant that helps move toxins from the lungs. It's also soothing to irritated lung tissues.
- **Oat seed or Oatstraw** help nourish and calm the nervous system while you're giving up tobacco.

You can also try mixing in other herbs with the tobacco, or substituting other herbs for the tobacco. (For Native Americans, the first tobacco smokers, tobacco comprised only about 5 to 10 percent of the blend of herbs that they smoked.) When you smoke these herbal mixtures, make it a ritual. Offer the smoke first in prayer and to the four directions.

Other herbs that are less harmful than tobacco and may be helpful to smoke during the transition period include:

Arnica flowers	Hawthorn leaves	Sarsaparilla
Buckbean	Lavender	Thyme
Burdock leaf	Licorice	Uva ursi
Catnip	Lobelia	Wood betony
Chamomile	Marjoram	Woodruff
Chervil	Mullein	Yarrow
Coltsfoot	Pearly everlasting	Yellow clover
Cornsilk	Red clover	Yerba santa
Damiana	Rosemary	
Eyebright	Sage	

Those who have been smoking mentholated tobacco may benefit from adding a bit of peppermint to the mixture.

❦ Smoker's Cough Tea ❧

This tea will relieve that hacking, persistent cough that troubles so many smokers.

1 cup water
1 teaspoon flaxseeds
1 teaspoon honey
1 teaspoon lemon

Bring the water to a boil. Stir in the flaxseeds and cover. Reduce the heat and simmer 15 minutes, then strain. Stir in the honey and lemon and drink.

Vitamin Therapy

A healthy diet is of utmost importance to a healthy lifestyle, and it becomes even more important when you're attempting to beat an unhealthy addiction like smoking. After years of smoking, your body is nutritionally unbalanced. Supplements can help you make a full recovery.

SUPPLEMENT	DOSAGE	COMMENTS
Vitamin C	500 mg every couple of hours	Take during the first few days of withdrawal to aid in detoxification and reduce nicotine cravings. Reduce the dosage gradually as your body recovers.
Vitamin A	10,000 IU three times daily	Helps strengthen the mucous membranes of the lungs.
Calcium-magnesium	1,000 mg calcium and 500 mg magnesium daily	These two supplements work best when combined in one pill. They'll help nourish and calm the nervous system.
B-complex vitamins	100 mg daily	Help nourish and calm the nervous system. B_1, B_6, and B_{12} help minimize cellular damage caused by tars and nicotine. Niacin helps widen the blood vessels and aids in the removal of lipids clinging to arterial walls, counteracting the effects of nicotine.
Zinc	25 mg daily	The body requires zinc to displace the cadmium that smoking deposits in the lungs Most smokers are zinc deficient Be sure the supplement is chelated zinc.
Vitamin E	400 IU daily	Vitamin E helps reduce cancer risk.

SUPPLEMENT	DOSAGE	COMMENTS
Selenium	200 mcg daily	Selenium helps reduce cancer risk and decreases sensitivity to cadmium, of which smoking leaves deposits on lung walls.
Tyrosine	1,000 mg twice daily	Take one dose in the morning and one dose in the afternoon to help curb cravings.
GABA (gamma-aminobutyric acid)	750 mg one to three times daily	GABA is a very calming amino acid that relieves anxiety.
L-glutamine	500 mg up to four times daily	Helps curb the blood sugar highs inherent to tobacco addiction.
L-cysteine	500 mg up to three times daily	Helps liquefy and expectorate mucus, reduces smoker's cough, and protects the lungs against both cadmium and acetaldehyde (one of the noxious chemicals found in cigarette smoke).

Hydrotherapy

Stay wet. You can't smoke very well when enjoying diversions such as swimming, showers, or long soaks in the bathtub. In addition, breathing in steam can help loosen old debris in the lungs.

Aromatherapy

Helichrysum aids tobacco detoxification, and black pepper essential oil helps alleviate nicotine withdrawal symptoms. Lemon, lime, grapefruit, and orange are other essential oils that can be used in aromatherapy to alleviate the desire for a smoke. Whenever you feel a strong craving, open a bottle of one of these essential oils and take a few deep breaths from the bottle.

Burn some dried artemesia or sage as incense. These herbs have long been used in sacred ceremonies. Surround yourself with their comforting, purifying smoke, rather than the polluting smoke of

**The Cure for
the Common Cold?**

I've known folks who a got
respiratory cold when they quit
smoking. They felt better when
they had a cigarette, so they
thought that smoking was the
cure. Not so! Once they stopped
smoking, all the particulate
matter and mucus that had
been accumulating in their
lungs was released. The cold
symptoms were simply a side
effect of the elimination process.

chemically cured tobacco. Breathe in the healing smoke. Say a prayer.

Nicotine Replacements

Nicotine gum, patches, and nasal sprays are all available techniques for giving up smoking. Ideally, you should use them for no more than a couple of months, though some continue their use for a year or longer. But this book is so full of natural alternatives that you should consider nicotine replacements a last resort. Pregnant women and those with ulcers or cardiovascular disease should avoid these alternative nicotine treatments.

To Avoid Weight Gain
When Quitting Smoking

It's common for people who've quit smoking to gain weight. When you quit, your senses of smell and taste improve, so appetite is often regained. Nicotine also speeds up metabolism and stimulates the entire gastrointestinal tract, so you may find that once you've quit your metabolism slows down. Remember, though, that it's not stopping the tobacco habit that causes weight gain—it's what you choose to eat after you've quit, when you're breaking the physical and psychological habit of smoking.

When substituting a snack for a smoke, select low-calorie items such as raw vegetables and unbuttered popcorn. Celery and carrot sticks make good nibbles. Go for high fiber and low fat.

If you're having a hard time controlling your appetite, try taking 500 milligrams of the amino acid L-phenylalanine between meals up to three times daily; this substance can decrease appetite. See also chapter 5 for tips and advice on controlling food cravings. But most important, keep in mind that a few extra pounds is less of a health risk than smoking tobacco.

7

Getting Sober
Dealing with Alcoholism

We are a society well versed in the dangers of alcohol. MADD, SADD, AA—most of us are familiar with these acronyms, because these and other organizations have been running grassroots campaigns against alcohol abuse for many years. Yet the news media is filled with reports of the ongoing rise in binge drinking, the younger and younger ages at which our children first start drinking, and the terrible tragedies caused by drunk driving. If we know that alcohol has such serious side effects, why are we still drinking?

Alcohol is an integral part of the social milieu of our culture, as it has been for centuries. It relaxes the body, loosens our inhibitions, and helps us feel sociable—less tense and more open to our emotions. But don't consider this an endorsement for drinking. For many of us, the risks inherent to drinking far outweigh any benefits. In the United States alone, there are more than ten million alcoholics, and alcoholism causes about two hundred thousand deaths a year.

Drinking doesn't necessarily mean that you're an alcoholic, of course. But if you find that one drink *always* leads to another, that you regularly say or do things while drinking that you later wish you hadn't, that you frequently suffer from blackouts, or that your drinking has caused arguments or tension between you and your family and friends, it may be time to take a good hard look at your relationship with alcohol.

The Chemistry of Drunkenness

Ethanol, the intoxicating agent in alcohol, is composed of tiny water-soluble molecules that affect every organ and nerve system of the body within minutes of ingestion. Ethanol is a simple sugar. When ingested, it passes through the stomach and intestines into the bloodstream and then on to the liver, where it's metabolized, or broken down. The liver can metabolize only a certain amount of alcohol per hour, regardless of the amount consumed. Excess alcohol remains in the bloodstream. When that excess ethanol reaches the central nervous system, it decreases brain activity and impairs physical coordination, speech, and the reflex system.

Red grape juice also contains many of the beneficial compounds found in wine.

Liquor	Alcohol Content
Beer	4%
Brandy	35–50%
Champagne	12–13%
Fortified wine (port, sherry)	17–20%
Gin	35–50%
Liqueur	20–50%
Rum	35–50%
Vodka	35–50%
Whiskey	Up to 50%
Wine	12–20%

Is Social Drinking Dangerous?

Many people can safely enjoy alcohol in moderate amounts. *Moderate drinking* is generally defined as no more than one drink—twelve ounces of beer, five ounces of wine, or an ounce and a half of 80-proof hard liquor—per day for women, and no more than two drinks a day for men.

Why are there separate guidelines for men and women? Studies have shown that when drinking equivalent measures of alcohol, women become more intoxicated than men, in part because their bodies do not break down alcohol as fast as men's bodies, so a larger percentage of the alcohol reaches the bloodstream. Also, women's bodies contain a smaller percentage of water than men's bodies, so that the alcohol remains more highly concentrated.

Alcohol's actions on the body are anesthetic, depressant, diuretic, euphoric, sedative, and soporific. In moderate amounts alcohol can stimulate the appetite, improve digestion, enhance cardiovascular function, improve circulation, and reduce the risk of heart attack. Alcohol drunk in moderation can elevate levels of the "good" cholesterol, or high-density lipoprotein (HDL), which can help prevent heart disease. Several studies have determined that moderate drinkers are less likely to develop heart disease than heavy drinkers or those who do not drink at all.

For those who drink without moderation, however, alcohol can be a serious health threat. In addition to the dangers inherent to the accidents and mishaps that accompany drunkenness, alcohol in large amounts increases your risk for heart disease, stroke, high blood pressure, liver cirrhosis, and, some studies suggest, cancer.

Drinking and Temperament

According to Danna Cunningham and Andrew Ramer, authors of *Further Dimensions of Healing Addictions,* what kind of alcohol someone is addicted to can tell us a lot about the drinker's temperament:

- **Beer** drinkers often have excess physical energy they aren't using. They should seek out physically and mentally stimulating activities.
- **Wine** imbibers are said to have excess mental energy and could benefit from more physical activity to get them out of their heads and more into their bodies. Or they could use that mental energy productively to write or pursue the arts.
- **Hard liquor** consumers tend to have excess emotional energy. They need to find constructive ways of expressing their emotions such as journaling, art, or therapy.

The Making of an Alcoholic

Next to sugar addiction (see chapter 3), alcoholism is the oldest and most prevalent addiction in America. It's estimated that 10 percent of men and 3 percent of women suffer from persistent problems related to alcohol abuse. Research has shown that alcoholism has a genetic marker: children of alcoholics are much more likely than the general population to develop alcoholism, even when they're removed at an early age from the alcoholic home. But there are many other factors, including sugar dependency, allergies, and the chemical reactions of the body, that contribute to the making of an alcoholic.

> **Warning**
>
> Anyone taking prescription drugs, women who are pregnant or soon planning to be, and people with diabetes, heart disease, hypertension, arthritis, gout, neuralgia, psoriasis or rosacea, yeast overgrowth, stomach disorders, liver ailments, chronic fatigue, and viral diseases should avoid alcohol altogether.

Alcohol addiction is at heart a sugar dependency. Low blood sugar is a factor for about 95 percent of alcoholics, and hypoglycemia may well be a major cause of alcoholism. Alcohol is the ultimate refined carbohydrate, capable of elevating blood sugar levels even faster than white sugar. Consuming alcohol gives a temporary rise in blood sugar so the imbiber feels relaxed and energized. When blood sugar drops, the desire to drink more rises. Over time an alcoholic may begin to consume alcohol in place of food, which causes even worse hypoglycemia.

Food allergies can also contribute to alcoholism. As described in chapter 5, food allergies or sensitivities often create food cravings; counterintuitively, the body often craves what it's allergic to. Many people allergic to yeast, wheat, barley, rye, or corn may find themselves craving an alcohol derived from that substance; consuming a beverage containing the offending substance fuels the allergy, creating a cycle of dependence.

Alcoholism can also be affected by malfunctioning chemistry in the body. Acetylaldehyde, the chemical produced by the liver as it metabolizes alcohol, is highly toxic and generally considered a carcinogen. In healthy people acetylaldehyde is quickly broken down, but alcoholics either produce excess acetylaldehyde or destroy it more slowly. When acetylaldehyde reaches the brain, it combines with neurotransmitters to form tetrahydroisoquinoline (THIQ), which causes a craving for alcohol and, like the drugs morphine and heroin, binds to the same receptor sites as naturally occurring endorphins.

Alcohol's Progeny: Liver Cirrhosis and Diabetes

Alcohol is a factor in a host of chronic and debilitating health conditions, including suppressed immune system, cancer, stroke, brain hemmorhage, sexual dysfunction, fetal alcohol syndrome, rosacea, premature aging, and many, many more. However, the two most common and deadly conditions alcoholism creates are cirrhosis of the liver and diabetes.

Cirrhosis of the liver is one of the most common and best-known side effects of alcoholism. When the liver cannot keep up with rate of alcohol being ingested, the unmetabolized alcohol kills liver cells and deposits fat in the liver. If alcohol consumption persists, damaged liver cells are replaced by scar tissue. As liver cirrhosis (scarring)

Eastern Perspectives on Alcoholism

Traditional Chinese medicine considers alcoholism to be a damp heat condition and alcohol to be a hot, damp, pungent, and ascending substance. Alcoholics are stuck in a cycle of relieving and then re-creating stagnant liver chi: alcohol's pungent taste can move stagnant liver chi, but its high sugar content impairs digestion and causes damp heat, which ultimately causes chi to stagnate in the liver again.

In Ayurvedic medicine alcohol is thought to heat the body; damage the liver, ojas, and blood; and increase Vata and Pitta. Kapha and Vata types are likely to be addicted to the sugar aspects of alcohol. Late stages of alcoholism are a Vata state—blank stare, shuffling gait, talkativeness without meaning, and delirium.

advances, the liver becomes less and less able to perform its many functions, which include filtering bacteria from the blood, storage and manufacturing of vitamins and nutrients, regulation of cholesterol and fats, regulation of metabolism, removal of waste products from the bloodstream, and metabolization of alcohol, to name just a few. When the liver can't perform, the body can't function. Cirrhosis

Alcohol causes the brain to deteriorate at a faster-than-normal rate; the brains of alcoholics are not usable by medical students studying anatomy because they have lost their structure and become mushy.

Women taking birth control pills are at even greater risk of developing cirrhosis from excessive alcohol consumption.

of the liver caused by alcoholism is one of the ten leading causes of death in the United States.

Alcoholism also contributes to many problems related to blood sugar levels, including, in serious cases, diabetes. For example, the liver is responsible for converting glucose (blood sugar) to glycogen (a form of glucose that can be stored in the liver). When the liver is persistently occupied with breaking down alcohol, it becomes less able to metabolize blood glucose and store it as glycogen. Excess sugar accumulates in the blood. The body tries to compensate by releasing extra insulin into the bloodstream, which lowers blood sugar levels. Later, when the body is in need of more blood sugar, the liver is unable to supply it and low blood sugar, also known as hypoglycemia, becomes a chronic problem. Low levels of glucose correspond to low levels of energy and impaired brain function. For temporary relief an alcoholic uses more alcohol, which contains plenty of sugar but serves only to exacerbate the problem.

Alcoholism can also cause hyperglycemia—too much sugar in the blood—for some people. The constant influx of alcohol creates persistent high blood sugar levels. As more and more insulin is released to compensate for the high blood sugar, the body becomes inured to its effects. Glucose intolerance and even diabetes can result.

Alcoholism Is Forever

There is no cure for alcoholism. A cure may never be found. An alcoholic who has been sober for a long time and has regained health must still avoid alcohol. Recovered alcoholics may no longer crave alcohol or suffer from withdrawal symptoms, but they may suffer relapses. If they drink again, they will most likely quickly find themselves addicted again. Numerous studies have shown that you cannot recover from alcoholism by cutting back. You must cut alcohol out of your life entirely.

Behavior Therapy

Giving up alcohol is, first and foremost, a change in consciousness. There is no magic pill you can take, no wonder drug that will overcome the alcohol dependency for you. If you are an alcohol abuser, the only force that can make you quit drinking is you. There are plenty of natural and herbal therapies that can help you through the withdrawal process, but they will not cure you. Only you can make that change.

You may fall off the wagon, as they say, a time or two. Most alcoholics trying to quit drinking do. But if you persevere; if you build a support network for yourself; and if you take things one day, or even one hour, at a time, you can and will overcome alcoholism.

For many alcoholics, fear is a motivating factor behind the desire to overcome alcoholism. They fear losing their family, their friends, their job, and their standing in the community. Ask for support from people in these networks. Tell your family and friends that you are quitting drinking—they will love you for it, and they will make every effort to help you. Find a support group, such as Alcoholics Anonymous, in your community. They're often listed in the yellow pages. Support groups are inexpensive and available worldwide. They have changed many people's lives for the better. Do whatever you can to find people, groups, and places that support you emotionally and spiritually.

While you're still in the withdrawal stage, avoid exposure to toxic chemical fumes such as those from cleaning fluids and gasoline. These can cause alcohol cravings in some people.

Throw out all the alcohol in your house. Practice your new nondrinking lifestyle just one day at a time. When you wake in the morning, tell yourself, *I will not drink today. Just today. I can get through this one day without alcohol.* Tell yourself this every day.

When you feel a craving for alcohol, practice relaxation or get some exercise. In addition, try some of the nutritional and herbal therapies discussed below.

Nutritional Therapy

When you quit drinking, it's essential that you feed your body a cleansing, healthy diet that supplies the nutrients it needs to recover from the degredations of alcohol abuse.

Remember that alcoholism is, at heart, a sugar dependency. You must be careful not to aid that dependency by giving the body the refined sugar it will crave. Research has shown that high-carbohydrate diets loaded with junk food tend to increase the desire for alcohol, while nutritious diets create less desire for alcohol. Alcoholics Anonymous recommends a high-protein, low-carbohydrate diet with nutritional supplements to help alcoholics stay sober. Good protein sources include fish, lean poultry, tofu, legumes, and nuts. Black soybeans are particularly nourishing and also help quell alcohol cravings. Tofu and mung beans have cooling and detoxifying properties that can help the body overcome alcoholism.

It's also important for a recovering alcoholic to keep the body's blood sugar level stable. Eat small, frequent meals. Avoid sugar, sweets, sweetened fruit juices, caffeine, and refined carbohydrates such as those found in breads and pasta. Eat plenty of vegetables and whole grains such as brown rice, oatmeal, millet, and buckwheat. Drink plenty of water, which will help cleanse the body and diminish cravings. To help detoxify the liver, add freshly squeezed lemon juice to your water.

When you have a craving for alcohol, try any of the following:

- **Dates** are nourishing and will satisfy your body's craving for something sweet.
- **Bananas, unsweetened fresh coconut, and Romaine lettuce** are said to deter alcohol desire.
- **Celery** helps balance the body's pH balance and is thought to lessen the desire for alcohol.

> When drinking juice to quiet the craving for alcohol, use a straw and drink as slowly as possible. Instead of feeding your addiction in one swift gulp, sipping slowly will help your body wean itself from its sugar dependency.

- **Tomato juice with lemon** squeezed into it is a popular folk remedy to ease the urge to drink.
- **Carrot juice** diluted by half with water will taste sweet enough to satisfy the body's sugar cravings and is cleansing to the liver.
- **Boysenberry juice** is another juice that tastes sweet and also decreases the desire for alcohol.
- **Fresh cabbage juice.** Cabbage contains small amounts of glutamine, which helps curb the brain's craving for alcohol. It's also helpful for alcoholics who have suffered liver and stomach distress.
- **Fresh string bean-and-tomato juice** is a semisweet juice that aids in repair of the liver.
- **Bitter tonic waters** will help dispel the craving for alcohol.

Herbal Therapy

Herbal therapy can help cleanse the body, relax the mind, and overcome alcohol addiction. Do not use alcohol tinctures; instead, use teas, glycerites, or capsules.

Cleansing herbs such as red clover blossoms, burdock root, and dandelion root can help detoxify the body. Also important will be calming nervines, such as oat seed or oatstraw and skullcap, to help you through the anxiety endemic to withdrawal. Liver tonics, such as alfalfa leaf,

Angelica flower essence can help you get to the root of an alcohol problem and aid in major life changes. Agrimony flower essence helps those who use alcohol or drugs to forget their pain.

ashwagandha, and bupleurum, will help your liver recuperate from alcohol abuse. Other herbs to try include the following:

- **Aloe vera** can help balance liver function and cool heat.
- **Angelica,** when used as capsules or tea, is said to help create a distaste for alcohol.
- **Chaparral** helps eliminate drug and alcohol residues from the body.
- **Cinnamon** is naturally sweet and thus satisfies the body's desire for sugar-rich alcohol. It also has a calming effect on the nerves.
- **Ginseng** nourishes the adrenal glands.
- **Gotu kola** helps detoxify the body and has a revitalizing effect on the nerves.
- **Kudzu flowers** have long been a remedy for drunkenness in traditional Chinese medicine. In studies done on alcoholic mice, when kudzu was consumed the mice decreased their alcohol consumption by 50 percent. It can be purchased in capsules. Kudzu root can also be used.
- **Milk thistle seed** capsules help prevent and repair alcoholic-induced liver disease.
- **Poria** helps to drain dampness.
- **St. John's wort** helps heal damaged nerves, lifts the spirits, and calms irritability.
- **Turmeric** improves liver function and protects the body from damage from alcohol.
- **Valerian** has sedative properties; try taking it in capsule form to help you get through the first few days of withdrawal.

Vitamin Therapy

Alcohol robs the body of nutrients, and alcoholics are commonly deficient in many vitamins and nutrients, especially vitamins A, B, and C, magnesium, and zinc.

Supplements to Help Overcome Alcoholism

SUPPLEMENT	DOSAGE	COMMENTS
Vitamin A	25,000 IU once daily	Helps revitalize the immune system.
B-complex vitamins	50 mg three times daily	A deficiency in B vitamins creates a greater need for glucose and inhibits liver function, which can contribute to alcohol cravings. In particular, thiamin (vitamin B_1) deficiency can contribute to confusion and memory loss. Niacin (vitamin B_3) helps prevent blood sugar levels from dropping, relieves anxiety, and, in conjunction with pantothenic acid, aids the breakdown of acetylaldehyde so it doesn't become THIQ.
Dimethlyglycine (DMG, B_{15}, or pangamic acid)	50–100 mg once a day for three weeks	Research has found that DMG causes many alcoholics to be indifferent to alcohol.
Vitamin E	400 IU twice daily	When combined with selenium, vitamin E helps prevent alcohol-induced lipoperoxidation, or free-radical damage.
Vitamin C	1,000 mg three times daily	Vitamin C is one of the most essential nutrients for detoxifying from addictions. It can reduce cravings, help detoxify the liver and blood, and nourish the adrenal glands.
Calcium	1,000 mg daily	Antispasmodic, sedative.
Magnesium	500 mg daily	Can help reduce the anxiety, restlessness, and delirium tremens that often accompany withdrawal.

SUPPLEMENT	DOSAGE	COMMENTS
Zinc	25 mg once a day	Zinc is essential to the detoxification of alcohol; a zinc deficiency makes the alcoholic more prone to liver cirrhosis.
Chromium (GTF)	200–400 mcg daily	Stabilizes blood sugar levels.
Selenium	200 mcg daily	Helps protect the liver from being damaged by alcohol.
L-glutamine	500 mg four to five times daily	Reduces alcohol cravings. For maximum effectiveness, take dosages between meals and at bedtime.
L-carnitine	300 mg three times daily	Helps the liver metabolize fatty acids, and helps reverse fatty liver disease induced by excessive alcohol consumption.
Tyrosine	1 g three times daily	Helps minimize stress, anxiety, and withdrawal symptoms.
Phosphatidylcholine	500 mg three times daily	To improve liver and brain function
Flaxseed or hempseed oil	1 tbsp. daily	Supplies essential fatty acids, which can reduce alcohol cravings, help restore brain and liver function, and minimize withdrawal symptoms.
Raw adrenal tablets	1 tablet twice daily	The adrenal glands tend to be exhausted after long-term substance abuse. Raw adrenal can help build strength when the body is depleted and exhausted.
Taurine	500 mg daily	Gradually reduce the dosage over several weeks to just 50 mg. Taurine can lessen or prevent withdrawal symptoms.

Aromatherapy

Aromatherapy can be a powerful ally for someone trying to quit drinking. Inhalations of various essential oils can quell cravings and ease withdrawal symptoms.

- **Bergamot** calms anxiety, lifts depression, and has a generally encouraging effect on the psyche.
- **Clary sage** is relaxing and rejuvenating. It helps relieve tension, fear, and paranoia and has a revitalizing effect on the nervous system.
- **Eucalyptus citriodora** is mildly stimulating and helps calm feelings of emotional overload.
- **Fennel** has a sweet fragrance that helps dispel sugar-based cravings for alcohol. It also helps promote self-motivation.
- **Helichrysum** helps detoxify the body and relieves depression, stress, and nervous exhaustion.
- **Juniper** calms anxiety and helps soothe those who feel emotionally drained.
- **Lemon** is uplifting; it brightens your outlook and helps open the emotional heart.
- **Marjoram** is relaxing and comforting; it helps calm emotional cravings.
- **Rose** encourages love and patience; it relieves sorrow and depression and helps you feel more emotionally open.
- **Rosemary** uplifts the spirit, stimulates memory and brain function, and helps relieve anxiety.
- **Sandalwood** calms nervous tension and anxiety; it can help you feel less isolated and/or emotionally volatile.

Remedies for Hangovers

If you've ever suffered from a hangover, you probably deserved it. However, everyone is entitled to a few mistakes.

The drinks most likely to cause hangovers include bourbon, brandy, champagne, cognac, rum, rye, whiskey, and red wine; vodka, gin, and white wine are less likely to cause hangovers. In general, the less flavor a substance has, the less likely it is to cause a hangover. Mixing several kinds of drinks increases hangovers, as does mixing alcohol with carbonated beverages, which enter the system too quickly.

Hangovers are produced by dehydration and hypoglycemia. To prevent a hangover, eat before drinking. When the stomach is full, alcohol absorption is slowed. Eat oily foods such as cheese or nuts before drinking and starchy foods while drinking. Eat a snack of fruit, or drink some fruit juice, before going to bed—the natural sugars will help your body metabolize the alcohol faster. Drink lots of water to avoid getting dehydrated. Take a teaspoonful of honey or a 100-milligram B-complex vitamin before bed and again upon arising to help break down alcohol in the body.

To dispel a hangover, drink a glass of orange or tomato juice or a teaspoon of umeboshi plum paste stirred into a cup of hot water. Eat a few dates to elevate your blood sugar levels, which will help you feel closer to normal.

Best of all, learn from your mistakes. If whatever you did the night before gave you a hangover today, don't take things to that extreme again!

8

Just What the Doctor Ordered
Beating Addictions to Prescription Stimulants and Tranquilizers

In a world of stress, anxiety, insomnia, family pressures, red-eye airline flights, ten-hour workdays, three-hour traffic jams—heck, world hunger and global warming!—it's no surprise that so many of us find ourselves in need of stimulants and tranquilizers. So we drink coffee, tea, espresso, and caffeinated sodas, and we have our afternoon martinis and late-night whiskeys. These "uppers" and "downers" are not without fault—as you can read in chapters 4 and 7, caffeine and alcohol deplete the body of nutrients and have their own set of dependency issues. But some of us also use synthetic stimulants and tranquilizers. Perhaps they were prescribed to us by a physician to treat insomnia or to help us through an emotionally difficult time. Perhaps they belong to a friend or loved one who hopes to help us by sharing his or her pre-scription. But make no mistake about it—they are legal, yes, and they are often prescribed by a physician, but if prescription stimulants or sedatives are used for an extended period of time or are taken in large doses, they can cause an addiction so severe that it has been likened to heroin dependency.

It's no secret that prescription stimulants and sedatives are addic-tive and dangerous. Just read the label on the bottle. What's worri-some is that they're some of the most commonly prescribed drugs in the world—and among the most often abused.

Amphetamine Stimulants

Amphetamines were first synthesized in 1887, although their stimu-lant properties were not recognized until 1927. They were originally used in the treatment of asthma. Later, amphetamines were used to treat narcolepsy, to treat hyperactivity in children, to counteract the effects of depres-sants, and (to a lesser degree) to aid weight loss and relieve fatigue and depression. Dur-ing World War II American, British, Ger-man, Italian, and Japanese soldiers were given hundreds of millions of doses of amphetamines—even though fatal intoxica-tions occurred often—in lieu of war rations and to help the soldiers overcome depression and low spirits.

The Amphetamine Family
Amphetamine
Dextroamphetamine
Methamphetamine
Biphetamine
Methylphenidate

Amphetamines are central nervous system stimulants. They create a feeling of euphoria and offer the body more energy, alertness, and ability to concentrate. They are twenty times more intense than cocaine—but they're legal.

As stimulants, amphetamines have a variety of uses. They're often taken by those who need to stay awake and alert for extended periods of time, such as long-distance drivers and soldiers on active duty. Stu-dents often use amphetamines not only to help them stay awake for long nights of studying but also to help them concentrate. Ampheta-mines suppress appetite, so they're often prescribed to dieters. And they're even used in various forms to treat hyperactivity—although it may seem odd to give a stimulant to treat hyperactivity, it works. Many researchers are involved in studying this paradox.

However, amphetamines have many serious side effects, and they can be addictive. There's no questioning the fact that amphetamines are physically addictive; any physician who prescribes them to you will warn you of this danger. But amphetamines also create a self-perpetuating cycle of psychological addiction. When the amphetamine buzz wears off, depression and lethargy set in. The answer? More amphetamines. And amphetamines used for an extended period of time—overextending the capacities of mind and body—can cause inertia, loss of perception, and mental dullness. The answer? Sadly, it's too often more amphetamines.

Side effects of amphetamines include increased heart rate, elevated blood pressure, heart palpitations, sweating, dry mouth, headache, insomnia, diarrhea, tremors, hallucinations, sleeplessness, confusion, restlessness, and a general feeling of apprehension and anxiety. Chronic amphetamine users suffer from sore throats, headaches, eye deterioration, and fatigue. They can become irritable and unstable and are likely candidates for nervous breakdowns.

Tolerance to amphetamines develops rapidly, requiring that the user take larger and larger dosages to feel the effects. However, large amounts of amphetamines can elevate blood pressure enough to blow out blood vessels to the brain and cause a stroke. Overdose can cause convulsions, coma, and even death.

As you might assume, amphetamines taken during pregnancy pose high risk to the infant. Pregnant women should never take amphetamines except under the strict supervision of their physician.

Herbal Therapy

A number of herbs can help you kick a stimulant addiction. Some help rebuild a body that has been worn down through long-term stimulant use. Others are natural stimulants that can be used as temporary substitutes for their chemical counterparts.

- **Aniseed** stabilizes blood sugar levels and is a natural energy builder.
- **Asparagus root** calms emotional irritability. It's highly nutritive and can help rebuild kidneys injured from long-term stimulant use.
- **Atractylodes rhizome** increases energy and builds chi.
- **Cola nut** is a natural stimulant. It does contain caffeine, though, which has its own drawbacks.
- **Dandelion root** helps remove drug residue from the body by improving liver function.
- **Ephedra** is a natural stimulant and can be used as a temporary substitute for chemical stimulants. See the cautions in chapter 2 before using ephedra.
- **Fennel seed** stabilizes blood sugar levels, decreases the desire for stimulants, and is mildly energizing.
- **Ginkgo leaf** improves cerebral blood flow and lifts depression.
- **Ginseng root** helps repair adrenal glands harmed from stimulant use and nourishes a frazzled nervous system.
- **Gotu kola** is a nerve and brain restorative. It can help you feel mentally alert without stimulants.
- **Green tea** is another natural stimulant. Like cola nut, though, green tea contains caffeine.
- **Ho shou wu root** is a nerve restorative. It calms anxiety and gently builds energy.
- **Hyssop** calms hysteria and cleanses drug residue from the body.
- **Jujube date** nourishes the adrenal glands, calms anxiety and depression, and is gently energizing.
- **Lemon balm** helps calm the spirit and makes withdrawal easier. It's also a mild antidepressant.
- **Licorice root** stabilizes blood sugar levels and functions as an adrenal and chi tonic.
- **Marsh mallow root** helps soothe and rebuild a dry, deficient constitution, such as one burned out from chemical stimulants.
- **Milk thistle seed** helps rebuild a liver damaged by drug abuse.
- **Oat seed** or **Oatstraw** nourishes the nerves and diminishes the desire for drugs.

- **Peppermint leaf** is a mild stimulant that also promotes relaxation.
- **Reishi mushroom** calms the nerves, reduces anxiety, and helps repair damage from long-term stimulant use.
- **Schizandra berry** improves physical endurance, calms anxiety, and is a nerve restorative.
- **Valerian root** can help your body rest and recover from over-stimulation.
- **Yerba maté** is a gentle stimulant that is also rich in antioxidants and can relieve depression.

Supplement Therapy

Here are some supplements that can aid in withdrawal from amphetamines:

SUPPLEMENT	DOSAGE	COMMENTS
B-complex vitamins	100 mg daily	Help maintain nervous system health and proper brain function. Can help alleviate anxiety and depression.
Calcium	1,000 mg daily	Helps maintain regular nerve impulses and neuromuscular activity.
Magnesium	500 mg daily	Helps nerve and muscle impulse transmissions. Calms nervousness and irritability and can prevent muscle twitching, depression, and dizziness.
L-phenylalanine	500 mg three times daily	Together with tyrosine (below), helps in the synthesis of the neurotransmitters dopamine and norepinephrine, which are mood regulators. Also helps elevate moods, improve memory and learning, curb appetite, and decrease pain. Not to be used by those with phenylketonuria.

SUPPLEMENT	DOSAGE	COMMENTS
Tyrosine	500 mg three times daily	Helps in the synthesis of norepinephrine and dopamine Elevates moods, curbs appetite, and helps reduce stress, depression, and anxiety.
Lecithin	1–3 tbsps. daily	Nutritive; improves brain function and calms anxiety.

Aromatherapy

Essential oils to smell to deter stimulant cravings include bergamot, clove, geranium, grapefruit, lemon, lime, and orange. These essential oils relieve stress and fatigue, uplift the spirits, and act as gentle stimulants.

Energy the Natural Way

Read the section Overcoming Fatigue and Increasing Energy in chapter 10 for ideas on healthy ways to get going.

Sedatives

Sedating agents can be broken down into two categories: barbiturates and everything else. *Tranquilizer* is often used to describe any tranquilizing agent that is not a barbiturate. For the sake of clarity, I will use *sedative* to describe all tranquilizing agents, including barbiturates, and *tranquilizer* to describe specifically nonbarbiturate sedating agents.

Sedatives are central nervous system depressants. They're often prescribed to reduce mental or physical tension, relieve anxiety, create a sense of well-being, relax the muscles, and cause drowsiness. In small doses they generally have a calming and relaxing effect on the central nervous system; in larger doses they induce sleep. When used over extended periods of time, however, they become highly addictive and can cause lethargy, irritability, nightmares, nausea, headache, skin rashes, impotence, and tremors.

Since the 1960s sedatives have been among the most abused drugs in the United States. Every year they're the drugs of choice for more than three thousand suicides and cause more than fifteen hundred accidental poisonings.

Using sedatives can slow your normal reactions, dull your feelings, and cause depression, appetite loss, dizziness, lethargy, speech problems, allergic reactions, digestive distress, constipation, diarrhea, headaches, menstrual and sexual disorders, sinus pain, joint pain, blurry vision, memory loss, and suicidal tendencies. As with alcohol, driving while under the influence of a sedative is dangerous. Sedatives impair both judgment and fine motor skills. If you're taking sedatives, under no circumstances should you be driving!

Barbiturates

Barbiturates are synthetic sedatives derived from barbituric acid. Barbiturates were first introduced in 1846 and were widely marketed from 1912 until about 1960, when nonbarbiturate sedatives replaced them. They're often prescribed to people with insomnia or excessive anxiety. However, they also have an effect that can be likened to an alcohol high—loss of inhibition, boisterous or aggressive behavior, loss of muscle coordination, and sedation—and so they have become common drugs of abuse.

The Name Game

- **Barbiturates** include amobarbital, aprobarbital, barbital, butabarbital, mephobarbital, methaqualone, methohexital, pentobarbital, phenobarbital, secobarbital, thiamylal, and thiopental.

- **Tranquilizers** are too numerous to list, but among them are chloral hydrate, chlordiazepoxide, ethclorvynol, flurazepam, glutethimide, hydroxyzines, lithium preparations, meprobamate combinations, methyprylon, molindone hydrochloride, nitrazepam, and thioxanthene.

- **Benzodiazepines** are a major class of nonbarbiturate tranquilizers. They include alprazolam, chlordiazepoxide, clonazepam, diazepam, estazolam, flurazepam, halazepam, lorazepam, midazolam, oxazepam, prazepam, quazepam, temazepam, and triazolam.

Barbiturates are extremely addictive; their physical and psychological habituation is considered as serious as that of heroin. They cause many accidental overdoses, because a toxic dose of barbiturates is often little more than what's needed to produce the

Never drink alcohol while you are taking sedatives. Alcohol multiplies a sedative's effect and can lead to accidental overdose—that is, coma or death. In addition, do not take sedatives if you are pregnant.

Impairment of judgment and fine motor skills will long outlast the sedative effects of a dose of barbiturates. You may feel that the dose has worn off before the effects have truly dissipated.

intoxicating effect. Following chronic high dosages, withdrawal symptoms can be extremely serious, even life threatening. They include insomnia, anxiety, tremors, convulsions, delirium, shock, and, in cases of abrupt withdrawal, coma and death.

Tranquilizers

Nonbarbiturate and benzodiazepine tranquilizers are generally safer than barbiturates, and consequently they are now the preferred drug for treatment of insomnia and anxiety. As the number of these sedatives available has risen—Americans take more than five billion a year—so, too, has the frequency of abuse and addiction.

Tranquilizers are less potent sleep inducers than are barbiturates, and they're less likely to interfere with motor skills. When they were first marketed in the 1950s and 1960s, most people believed they were nonaddictive and perfectly safe to use. Research has since disproved this innocent theory.

Tranquilizers were originally used to treat psychoses, including schizophrenia; to calm violence and hyperactivity; and to make patients more receptive to therapy. Nowadays they're most often used to treat insomnia and stress. They're intended to be used for short periods only (from one to six weeks) to help people through difficult times, such as divorce or the death of a loved one. Most people can give them up without problems after these short periods of usage, though about 25 percent of users encounter withdrawal reactions.

When tranquilizers are used for extended periods of time, they begin to lose their beneficial effects, and they become more difficult to give up. Users will develop a tolerance and must take more to produce any effect, leading to an accelerated rate of dependency and possible overdose.

If you have used tranquilizers, including benzodiazepines, for more than four weeks straight, withdraw gradually rather than quitting cold turkey, and consult with your physician for advice first. Abrupt withdrawal can cause nausea, cramps, delirium, convulsions, and in rare cases sudden death.

Benzodiazepine tranquilizers are the most commonly prescribed of nonbarbiturate sedatives. They're generally safe for short-term use (though they become potentially lethal when combined with alcohol); still, when used for extended periods of time they can become addictive.

Benzodiazepines slow heartbeat and respiratory rate, lower blood pressure, and have a mildly depressing action on the nervous system. They often cause loss of coordination and dizziness. They can also induce sleep, though they decrease the amount of REM dream time and inhibit the emotional clearing that is a vital function of dreaming and sleeping. When benzodiazepines are discontinued, they can have a rebound effect marked by vivid and excessive dreams.

Behavior Therapy

Because sedatives have an effect similar to that of alcohol, follow the guidelines for alcohol addiction outlined in chapter 7. Sudden withdrawal from sedatives is very dangerous; it traumatizes the liver and heart and can cause seizures, coma, or even death. Daily doses are best decreased gradually—by 10 to 25 percent every week or month, depending on how large your average dose is. The longer you've been taking sedatives, the slower the letting-go process should be.

If you're using sedatives originally prescribed by a physician, consult with him or her about decreasing their use. Those suffering from a strong addiction to barbiturates or tranquilizers should undergo the withdrawal process in a clinically supervised setting.

Herbal Therapy

There are many herbs that can benefit someone struggling to give up an addiction to prescription sedatives.

- **Ashwagandha** helps rebuild a nervous system depleted by drug use. It calms anxiety, stress, and tremors and reduces mental fatigue.

- **Atractylodes** increases energy, builds chi, and helps restore a liver damaged by drug abuse.
- **Blue vervain** is a mild sedative; it relieves insomnia and calms anxiety.
- **Bupleurum** is a mild muscle relaxant. It helps mellow anger and relieve depression, stress, and pain.
- **Calamus** calms hysteria, relieves depression, and enhances perception. It helps restore brain function that has been impaired by drug abuse.
- **California poppy** is a safe, natural sedative that calms restlessness and anxiety.
- **Catnip** is a mild sedative that calms anxiety and restlessness.
- **Chamomile flowers** relieve anxiety, insomnia, pain, and stress and can decrease nightmare episodes.
- **Codonopsis root** helps relieve insomnia and stress while also improving energy levels.
- **Corydalis** is an effective pain-relieving agent that is nonaddictive.
- **Cyperus** is a natural sedative. It's especially helpful during the withdrawal period.
- **Ginseng** nourishes the nerves and adrenal glands. It helps relieve stress and improves physical and mental energy.
- **Gotu kola** is a nerve and brain restorative that also improves depression.
- **Hops** are a natural sedative that relieve anxiety, stress, and insomnia. Hops can also calm delirium and tremors that may occur during withdrawal.
- **Jujube dates** calm the spirit and replenish depleted adrenal glands and nerves.
- **Kava kava** calms fear, pain, and anxiety. It's mildly euphoric and can encourage deep, restful sleep.
- **Lavender flowers** ease the withdrawal from sedatives. Lavender is itself a natural sedative and can calm and lift the spirits.
- **Lemon balm** also eases the withdrawal from sedatives. It's mildly mood elevating yet also calming.
- **Licorice root** helps stabilize blood sugar levels, relieves stress and fatigue, and promotes calmness.

- **Linden leaf and flower** calm the spirits and reduce stress and anxiety.
- **Lobelia** tincture can be given as an antispasmodic, especially in cases of muscle spasms.
- **Milk thistle seed** improves the breakdown and release of drug residues stored in the liver.
- **Motherwort** calms anxiety and hysteria; it functions as both a sedative and a rejuvenative.
- **Mugwort** can be used in small amounts to help the body detoxify. It also calms hysteria and lifts depression.
- **Oat seed or Oatstraw** decreases anxiety and calms and strengthens the nerves. Both help decrease the desire for sedatives.
- **Passionflower** helps relieve stress and insomnia. During the withdrawal period it can calm and comfort the spirit.
- **Reishi mushroom** relieves stress, anxiety, and insomnia by calming the nerves.
- **Sage** clears drug residues from the body and restores the nerves.
- **St. John's wort** helps lift the depression and anxiety that may be the root cause of addictive tendencies.
- **Schizandra berry** calms anxiety, relieves irritability, and is a nerve restorative.
- **Skullcap** calms anxiety and relaxes tremors during withdrawal.
- **Valerian root** can be used as a nonaddictive alternative for sedatives. It aids sleep and relaxes the muscles.
- **Wood betony** relieves anxiety and is a nerve restorative.

Supplement Therapy

The following supplements can aid in withdrawal from sedatives:

SUPPLEMENT	DOSAGE	COMMENTS
Calcium	1,000 mg daily	Can help prevent muscle cramps and spasms; aids sleep and raises the pain threshold.
Magnesium	500 mg daily	Can relieve fatigue, mental confusion, and irritability and reduce muscle cramps.
B-complex vitamins	100 mg daily	Improve brain and nerve function, decrease mental confusion and irritability, and improve the attention span.
Vitamin C	1,000 mg eight times daily	Aids in the detoxification process. After a few weeks, gradually decrease the number of dosages to just once daily. If diarrhea occurs, use less.
DLPA	500 mg four times daily	DLPA is a form of the amino acid phenylalanine, which aids in the production of norepinephrine and slows the breakdown of natural endorphins and enkephalines, which in turn help reduce pain perception. DLPA is not to be used by anyone with phenylketonuria.

A pilot study conducted by Alfred Libby and Irwin Stone (as cited by Ruth Long in the 1989 edition of *The Official Nutrition Education Association Home Study Course in the New Nutrition*) examined the use of vitamin C in giving up addictions. Drug addicts were given sodium ascorbate, a form of vitamin C that's easy on the digestive tract. The greater the amount of drugs they'd used, the higher the dose of vitamin C they received. The researchers found that the vitamin seemed to minimize withdrawal symptoms. After a few days the addicts reported restored appetite, restful sleep, and a genuine sense of feeling good.

Aromatherapy

Inhalations of the following essential oils can be very effective in helping you overcome an addiction to sedatives:

- **Chamomile** relieves tension, quiets anger and oversensitivity, and aids sleep.
- **Geranium** lifts depression, relieves stress, and makes you feel more mentally alert.
- **Jasmine** helps relieve fear, pessimism, and depression and boosts self-confidence.
- **Lavender** is cleansing and emotionally balancing. It helps relieve stress and insomnia, soothes anger, and lifts depression.
- **Marjoram** dispels grief, anxiety, irritability, and insomnia.
- **Neroli** is a natural antidepressant. It's calming and relaxing and helps relieve anxiety, fear, hopelessness, and depression.
- **Rose** helps you feel more loving and patient. It relieves grief and depression.

Natural Ways to Conquer Stress, Insomnia, and Anxiety

Addiction to sedatives is often a consequence of stress, insomnia, and anxiety. For information on natural methods for dealing with stressors, turn to chapter 10.

PART THREE

When You've Finally
Decided to Quit

9

Jitterbug Blues
Making It through the Withdrawal Period

If you've made the decision to kick your addiction, congratulations! A happier, healthier world is awaiting you. First, though, you have to get through the withdrawal period. Many people have multiple addictions, and you may find it easier to tackle the most serious of them first—alcohol before tobacco and tobacco before chocolate, for example—but following the program for one addiction may well put you on the road to recovery for others as well. If you are eating a healthier diet and supporting your body with herbs and supplements, you may find that by the time you have dealt with the more serious addictions, the others have almost resolved themselves.

For some people, withdrawal symptoms don't amount to much, while for others they pose a serious challenge. And withdrawal is more than simply enduring cravings for a particular substance; you may feel jittery, irritable, or depressed, and you may have physical symptoms ranging from headaches to tremors.

For many, the distress of withdrawal serves as an incentive to stay addiction-free. They don't want to have to go through that again! And withdrawal can be a real awakening—if you thought that your addiction wasn't all that serious, the symptoms of withdrawal can show you just how much your body depended on that chemical substance.

It can take a year or more before you feel completely healed physically and stable emotionally. But it's well worth it! The road to recovery brings you revitalized energy, health, and happiness. You'll feel better, look better, and live better. All you have to do is make the decision—and stick with it!

Detoxification

Addictive substances disrupt the body's normal processes and the mind's normal thought patterns. To kick an addiction, you must detoxify both body and mind, first by cleansing, and then by rebuilding.

- **Cleansing** means avoiding the substance of your addiction; drinking teas and eating foods that help cleanse the body of toxic wastes and drug residue; and giving up the psychological dependency.
- **Rebuilding** involves supporting and nurturing those bodily organs and systems that have been weakened or damaged by the addiction; learning new, healthier habits that can replace the unhealthy behavior of addiction; and building networks of emotional support to help you through the withdrawal period.

Physiological effects from substance abuse are almost always reversible. But when you make the decision to free yourself from an addiction, your body does not return to its natural state overnight. Have patience.

Withdrawal Symptoms

Symptoms of withdrawal are many, and occurrence and severity vary from person to person. Symptoms can include sweating, nausea, diarrhea, constipation, difficulty in breathing, body aches, chills, shaking, sensitivity to light and touch, headaches, heart palpitations, anxiety, confusion, depression, panic, hallucinations, paranoia, and rage. Withdrawal from severe cases of alcoholism or barbiturate addiction can cause delirium tremens, a sometimes violent state of mental disorder characterized by confusion, disordered speech, and hallucinations accompanied by tremors.

> The shaking of the body that characterizes delirium tremens is what gave rise to the term *kicking the habit.*

Symptoms of withdrawal usually occur twenty-four to seventy-two hours after the last dose of a substance. The most dramatic symptoms abate after five to seven days, but the entire process can last anywhere from a few days to a few months. Irritability and sleeping disorders can endure even longer.

Gradual withdrawal is recommended over quitting cold turkey. A slow and steady withdrawal may prolong the discomfort, but it's both safer and easier, and in the long run it produces fewer side effects.

Be Open with Family and Friends

Beating an addiction is hard work, and you're most likely to be successful if you have the help of those who love you.

If you live alone, ask a relative or close friend to spend the first few days with you. Let the people you live with and work with know what you're doing. Ask them not to take personally any emotional outbursts you may have over the next few days. Tell them that your irritability and changeable mood will be temporary.

Understanding what's occurring makes the withdrawal process easier. Try talking with friends or family who have been

When to Seek More Help

In some cases withdrawal from an addiction is best undertaken in a controlled medical environment. If you have a history of grand mal seizures, heart problems, or psychiatric problems, or if you have a serious addiction to alcohol or sedatives, you should undertake the detoxification process in a hospital. In addition, if you begin your withdrawal at home and experience any of the following, consult with your primary health care provider for advice:

- Delirium tremens, or the "shakes"
- The onset of illness that seems more serious than the flu
- Severe depression

through a similar withdrawal process. Ask them how it went for them, and what they did to get through the withdrawal period. Commiserating together, you may find added strength to endure the symptoms of withdrawal and overcome the addiction.

Behavior Therapy

The process of cleansing your body offers an excellent opportunity to clean house—literally. Get rid of clutter. Clean out the cobwebs. Organize. Unwanted clutter in the house can be a symbol of unwanted clutter in the body—your addiction. Get rid of it!

Journaling can be very helpful when you're facing a craving. Write about what you're experiencing, both physically and emotionally. Draw pictures to accompany the words.

> Do not mistake a withdrawal symptom for an anxiety attack, bout of depression, or severe insomnia. Whatever comes up during the withdrawal process, be willing to learn from it and resolve it.

Reward yourself for targeted amounts of success. After a day—or a morning or an hour—take a soothing warm bath, drop money in a "buy-yourself-something-nice" savings jar, or do whatever else you find enjoyable.

Use the withdrawal time as a period for rest. Large-print books of light subject matter and easy crossword puzzles can be a mild diversion. Calming music can help soothe the spirit.

Crying cleanses the body, mind, and soul. Allow it to happen.

Sound Therapy

Sound can be a powerful ally in releasing old "stuck" emotions and programming. Lie on your back with your mouth open and make a long *ahhhh* sound as you exhale. Give a sound to the feeling of addiction. If a sound isn't coming spontaneously, then tone low and slow and gradually raise the pitch until it vibrates with the pain. Continue making sounds until you feel a release. Feel that as the sound leaves your body, it's bringing out with it old pain, debris, and stuckness. Then breathe in positive energy.

Practice this for no more than three minutes at a time, but repeat it two to four times daily.

Exercise

Exercise stimulates endorphin release, encourages better use of oxygen, and relaxes the mind. Stretching, yoga, gardening, deep-breathing exercises, and other forms of light, relaxing movement are all recommended during the initial withdrawal period. You can also use exercise as a symbol of the process you're undergoing: Fling your arms, body, and head in a way that signifies throwing off or being rid of. Shake your body.

Skin Brushing

Skin is often referred to as the third lung, and dry-brushing the skin can aid in the detoxification of the body by boosting circulation and improving lymphatic flow. As a side benefit, after regular practice you'll end up with soft, glowing, healthy skin.

Skin brushing should be done with a soft vegetable-fiber brush just before you bathe. Disrobe and, starting with your feet, gently brush the skin in a circular motion. Work your way up the legs, then the hands and arms, and finally the torso, both front and back. The entire procedure should take two to three minutes. Be especially gentle over the breasts and avoid the genitals. Then shower or bathe. End with cool water to give yourself a forced circulatory massage.

Every two weeks wash the brush and dry it in the sun or a warm place.

Hydrotherapy

Soaking in a tepid bath to which three pounds of Epsom salts have been added is not only relaxing but also helps detoxify your system and draw out old drug and chemical residues. Neutral-temperature baths (between 92 and 98 degrees) soothe the nervous system and promote detoxification.

Sauna baths, sweat lodges, and steam baths also speed the release of toxic substances through sweating. They can have profoundly healing and spiritually opening effects if you enter them with the intention of releasing and purifying. They should, however, be enjoyed with a buddy, because the intense heat can lead to lightheadedness and dizziness.

After a detox bath or sweat therapy, rinse off, get covered up, and enjoy some bedrest. Those with high blood pressure should consult their doctor before using any bath or sweat therapies.

Nutritional Therapy

It's imperative to keep your blood sugar levels stable during the detoxification process. Unstable blood sugar levels drain you of energy and can contribute to cravings. To stabilize blood sugar levels, eat four or five small meals a day. Have a healthy snack before bed and then eat again early in the morning.

Green leafy vegetables provide ample amounts of vitamins, minerals, and fiber. Their high nutrient content nourishes the body and promotes regeneration of damaged systems, their chlorophyll helps the body better utilize oxygen, and their fiber content aids in the elimination of toxins.

High-sulfur vegetables such as broccoli, cabbage, and cauliflower also aid in detoxification. They are full of antioxidants, which help protect the body against free radicals.

To add more calming calcium to your diet, eat yogurt or drink goat's milk.

Protein is also important during withdrawal, because it can reduce cravings. Good protein sources include legumes, tofu, tempeh, poultry, nuts, seeds, and eggs. Fish is an excellent source of protein and is rich in the raw material the body needs to make its needed neurotransmitters.

Do not eat sugar—as a superrefined carbohydrate without much nutritional value, it will keep your body in an addictive mode, as I discussed in chapter 3. Reduce your intake of refined foods. Choose organic foods whenever possible.

Those who experience digestive distress during the withdrawal process may fare well to easy-to-digest foods such as high-protein baby food, blended soups, and pureed vegetables.

Be sure to drink plenty of pure water so that wastes may be more effectively carried away. Have a drink of water whenever a craving arises. The addition of a bit of lemon juice to the water you consume can be even more effective: its sour flavor stimulates liver cleansing. Diluted unsweetened cranberry juice is also cleansing to the liver and kidneys.

> To minimize shaking and tremors during withdrawal, eat adequate protein and plenty of whole grains such as oatmeal, millet, and brown rice.

If you experience diarrhea or vomiting, be sure to drink electrolyte-rich beverages to help rehydrate and replace lost trace minerals.

The following recipes are easy to prepare and pleasing to the palate. Each one combines several nutrient-dense foods that are of immense support to the body and mind during the withdrawal period.

❦ Detox Juice Mix ❧

This combination tastes great, is highly nutritive, and supports cleansing of the liver, kidneys, and colon.

1 part carrot juice
1 part beet juice
1 part celery juice
1 part wheat grass juice
1 part lime juice
5 parts pure springwater

Combine all ingredients and drink.

❦ Kudzu Cream ❧

Kudzu is a restorative tonic, helping nourish and soothe the body. It's easy to digest—especially helpful for those who have not been kind to their digestive systems—and strengthens intestinal weakness. It stabilizes blood sugar levels and has long been used as a traditional Chinese medicine remedy for those who consume too much alcohol and to counteract toxins.

1¼ cups water
1½ teaspoons kudzu powder
1 teaspoon tamari

Bring 1 cup of the water to a boil in a small pan. Dissolve the kudzu in the remaining ¼ cup water and add to the pan. Stirring constantly, bring to a boil. Reduce the heat and simmer for 2 to 3 minutes. Add the tamari. Makes 2 servings.

Variation: Use apple juice in place of the water. Omit the tamari.

֍ Carrot Ginger Soup ֍

Not only is this soup delicious, but it's also high in nerve-nourishing calcium and lung-strengthening beta-carotene. Carrots are considered one of the best detoxifying agents and are very effective in helping cleanse the liver and kidneys. This soup is easy to digest and will also improve circulation.

> **1 cup chopped onion**
> **3 cloves garlic**
> **1 tablespoon vegetable oil**
> **4 cups chopped carrots**
> **2 teaspoons grated ginger**
> **1½ teaspoons salt**
> **3 cups water**

Sauté the onion and garlic in the vegetable oil. Add the carrots, ginger, salt, and water. Simmer for 1 hour. Let the mixture cool a bit, then puree it in the blender. Return to the soup pot and reheat. Makes about 6 cups.

֍ Kitcheri ֍

Kitcheri is high in valuable protein and complex carbohydrates, which can reduce addictive cravings and ease withdrawal symptoms. It's easy to prepare and easy to digest. In Ayurvedic medicine kitcheri is said to purify both physical and mental toxins as well as improving the memory. In India people often eat nothing but kitcheri for a week or more at a time to cure a wide variety of ailments.

> **2 cups dried mung beans**
> **3 teaspoons coriander seeds**
> **1½ teaspoons whole cumin seeds**
> **8 cups water**
> **1½ cups long-grain brown rice**
> **2 tablespoons olive oil**
> **2 teaspoons ground turmeric**
> **Salt and pepper**

Rinse the beans and soak them overnight in water in the refrigerator. In the morning rinse them again. In a skillet roast the coriander and cumin over high heat, stirring constantly for about 3 minutes. Bring the water to a boil in a large covered pot and add the remaining ingredients. Simmer for about 1½ hours. Season with salt and pepper to taste.

☙ Carrot Rice Loaf ☙

This simple and tasty loaf combines the beta-carotene and calcium of carrots (which nourish the lungs and nervous system) with the B-complex vitamins and whole grains of brown rice (which enhance energy while calming the body). Almonds are considered a "building food"—excellent if you've eaten poorly for a long time—and they're easy to digest.

> ½ cup almond butter
> ½ cup raw sunflower seeds
> 4 cups cooked brown rice
> 4 cups grated raw carrots
> ½ cup coarse bread crumbs
> 1 onion, chopped and sautéed
> 1 teaspoon salt
> 1 tablespoon dried sage leaves

Mix the almond butter, sunflower seeds, and rice. Add the remaining ingredients and place into an oiled baking dish. Bake at 350 degrees for 45 minutes. Makes 6 servings.

☙ Roasted Roots ☙

Roots are naturally sweet and can help stabilize blood sugar levels to diminish cravings. They're cleansing to the liver and aid in the elimination of toxins from the body. This delicious dish combines a wide assortment of roots with tempeh—a soy product that provides protein as well as anxiety-calming lecithin—for a satisfying repast.

> 1 cup chopped carrots
> 1 cup chopped onion
> 1 cup chopped potatoes
> 1 cup peeled chopped sweet potatoes
> ½ cup peeled chopped rutabaga
> ½ cup peeled chopped beets
> 1 8-ounce package tempeh, sliced into 16 pieces

1 tablespoon olive oil
¼ cup water
2 tablespoons tamari
2 cloves garlic, minced
1 tablespoon fresh-grated gingerroot

Preheat the oven to 400 degrees. Place all the ingredients into a baking dish with a lid and stir. Cover and bake for 1 hour. Makes 4 to 6 servings.

❦ Congee ❦

Congee is a slow-cooked porridge that's easy to eat and digest. It's wonderful for those who haven't quite regained an appetite but have a high requirement for nutrients. This congee combines pungent herbs that improve circulation with barley, which strengthens a weak digestive system and soothes an irritated liver—both of which result from substance abuse. The jujube dates support exhausted adrenal glands and nourish the liver; they're uesd in Traditional Chinese medicine to calm the spirit.

1 inch fresh gingerroot, peeled and chopped
2 teaspoons dried cinnamon
1 teaspoon cardamom seeds, crushed (remove from
   pod if using whole seeds)
2 carrots, chopped
¾ cup lightly pearled barley
2 cups water
12 jujube dates, pitted

Mix all the ingredients in a large pot and simmer together for 2 hours. Makes 4 to 6 servings.

❦ Borscht ❦

Beets are one of nature's best internal cleansers, especially for the liver and bowels. They're high in iron and help build red blood cells, which can boost energy levels. Don't be alarmed if your stool is red for a few days after eating this borscht, because beet pigment often causes bodily wastes to be reddish. Beets are also naturally sweet, which stabilizes blood sugar levels and helps satisfy addictive cravings. The other main ingredients of borscht are also healing for the body: cabbage is rich in antioxidants, and potatoes provide calming complex carbohydrates.

1 tablespoon vegetable oil
1 onion, chopped

1 cup chopped cabbage
2 potatoes, chopped
4 medium beets, peeled and cut into pieces
5 cups water
$\frac{1}{2}$ teaspoon salt

Heat the vegetable oil in a soup pot and in it sauté the onion. Add the cabbage and stir, then add the potatoes and beets. Add the water, cover the pot, and simmer until the vegetables are tender. Puree half of the soup in a blender, then pour the puree back into the pot and stir. Season with salt. Makes 5 to 6 servings.

♦ Supersonic Tonic Smoothie ♦

This is a great way to start your day! Yogurt is rich in calcium, which calms the nerves, as well as in friendly bacteria to nourish the intestines. The remaining ingredients could all be described as superfoods: powerhouse supplies of nutrients crammed in small packages. Ginseng supports energy and willpower and helps revitalize exhausted adrenal glands. Flax- or hempseed oil provides essential fatty acids that can help deter cravings. Lecithin calms anxiety and improves mental alertness. Nutritional yeast is rich in calming yet energizing B vitamins and also contains protein. Almond butter is another good source of protein and B-complex vitamins. The blueberries are blood cleansing and laxative.

1 cup yogurt
1 peeled ripe banana
$\frac{1}{2}$ teaspoon ginseng powder
1 tablespoon flax- or hempseed oil
1 tablespoon lecithin
1 tablespoon nutritional yeast
1 tablespoon almond butter
$\frac{1}{4}$ cup frozen blueberries

Puree all the ingredients together in a blender and enjoy as a beverage.

❦ Bliss Balls ❦

This sweet treat is high in fiber, complex carbohydrates, and protein.
The oats support the nerves, and the sunflower seeds aid exhausted adrenals.
The warming spices enhance digestion. Raisins are definitely a sweet, but they
are also a laxative and are considered beneficial for the digestive tract, liver,
kidneys, and blood. Bliss Balls should not replace a meal, but they can
certainly replace that candy bar you're craving!

1 cup raw sunflower seeds
¹/₂ cup quick-cooking oatmeal
1 cup pumpkin seeds
¹/₂ cup carob powder
1 tablespoon bee pollen (optional)
¹/₂ teaspoon dried cinnamon
¹/₂ teaspoon dried cardamom
¹/₂ teaspoon powdered ginger
¹/₂ cup raisins
2 tablespoons almond butter
¹/₂ cup honey or maple syrup
1 teaspoon vanilla extract

In a large bowl place ¹/₂ cup of the sunflower seeds along with the oatmeal, pumpkin seeds, carob powder, bee pollen, cinnamon, cardamom, ginger, and raisins. In a separate bowl combine the almond butter, honey, and vanilla. Now mix the wet and dry ingredients together and stir. Form into ¹/₂-inch-diameter balls with your fingers and roll each ball into the remaining ¹/₂ cup of sunflower seeds. Store in the refrigerator for up to two weeks. Makes about 30 balls.

Herbal Therapy

Each of the previous chapters detailed herbs specific for particular addictions, whether you're wanting to eliminate refined sugar from your diet or give up smoking. The herbs listed here are specific for cleansing and rebuilding the body and mind. They can be of tremendous assistance during the withdrawal period.

- **Ashwagandha** lifts the spirits and relieves depression. It can help rebuild the nerves after the stress of addiction.

- **Bupleurum root** helps clear stored negative emotions from the liver. It also improves adrenal exhaustion.
- **Burdock root** helps the body clean out drug and alcohol residue.
- **Dandelion root** also helps remove drug and alcohol residues from the body.
- **Fennel seed** helps stabilize blood sugar levels, thereby reducing cravings for addictive substances.
- **Goldenseal root** can quickly remove drug residues from the kidneys, liver, and blood. Take 2 capsules three times daily. Use for only ten days. (Goldenseal is an endangered herb, so buy only cultivated, not wildcrafted, supplies.)
- **Kava kava rhizome** calms fear and anxiety and aids sleep.
- **Lavender flowers** lift the spirits and decrease the desire for addictive substances.
- **Lemon balm herb** is a nerve rejuvenative and can help lift the spirits.
- **Licorice root** helps stabilize blood sugar levels, which lessens addictive cravings. It can also help you feel more peaceful.
- **Oat seed or Oatstraw** lessens anxiety as well as the desire for addictive substances.
- **Passionflower** calms the spirit and makes you feel more restful.
- **Reishi mushroom** calms anxiety and aids sleep.
- **Siberian ginseng root** nourishes exhausted adrenal glands and nerves. It supports the body during times of change and stress.
- **Skullcap herb** eases anxiety and panic and can calm tremors.
- **Valerian root** aids sleep and calms anxiety. Take 2 capsules three times daily.
- **Yellow dock root** helps the body's natural cleansing process, especially in the kidneys and lymphs.

❧ Withdrawal Relief Tea ❧

This tea formula addresses the multiple tasks of treating withdrawal: cleansing drug residue from the body, stabilizing blood sugar levels, and relieving anxiety. You can make up your own tea formula by substituting for the herbs recommended here any herbs that you've found work better for you.

4 cups water
1 heaping teaspoon burdock root

> 1 teaspoon fennel seeds
> 1 teaspoon oat seed or oatstraw
> 1 teaspoon skullcap herb

Bring the water to a boil. Add the burdock root, reduce the heat, cover, and simmer over low heat for 15 minutes. Remove from the heat and add the remaining herbs. Cover and let steep for 10 minutes. Strain.

Drink 1 cup. Store the leftovers in the refrigerator, where they will keep for up to 3 days. Makes 4 cups.

Supplement Therapy

The previous chapters have detailed information on supplements helpful for treating particular addictions. The supplements listed here are more generally helpful: they lift the spirits, calm the mind, and help rejuvenate and rebuild the body.

Most of the supplements have a dosage range listed. Use the highest dosage for the first two weeks of withdrawal. Gradually decrease to a midrange dosage for the next three to six weeks, and then a normal or low dosage for the next few months.

SUPPLEMENT	DOSAGE	COMMENTS
B-complex vitamins	100 mg one to three times daily	Help maintain nerve health and proper brain function.
Lecithin	1 tbsp. one to three times daily	Calms anxiety.
Acidophilus	2 capsules three times daily	Helps restore friendly flora to the intestinal tract so that nutrients can be absorbed.
Vitamin C	1,000 mg every two to four hours	Take this dosage until cravings have ceased, then decrease the amount to twice daily. Vitamin C is one of the most essential nutrients for detoxifying from addictions. Buffered vitamin C is easiest on the stomach.

SUPPLEMENT	DOSAGE	COMMENTS
Flax- or hempseed oil	1–3 tbsps. or 2–6 capsules daily	A good source of essential fatty acids, which calm addictive cravings.
DHA (docosahexaenoic acid)	1,200 mg three times daily	Substance abuse depletes DHA from nerve tissue; a deficiency can contribute to depression, aggression, and impulsive behavior.
GTF chromium	200 mcg three to five times daily	Imperative to stabilize blood sugar levels. Helps reduce cravings.
Calcium	800–1,500 mg daily	Aids in neurotransmitter release and heartbeat regulation. Calms the nervous system and promotes sleep and rest.
Magnesium	400–750 mg daily	Helps stabilize blood sugar levels, relieves spasms, relaxes muscles, and calms nerves.
L-glutamine	250 mg three to four times daily	Helps stabilize blood sugar levels. To stop intense cravings, open a capsule and let the contents dissolve on your tongue.
Taurine	250–500 mg once or twice daily	Can help stop tremors associated with withdrawal.
GABA (gamma-aminobutyric acid)	750 mg daily	Calms the mind; minimizes excitatory messages to the brain.
5 HTP	100 mg two to three times daily	Helps relieve anxiety, depression, mood swings, excessive appetite, sugar cravings, and alcoholism.
Chlorophyll	1–3 capsules daily	Purifying and rejuvenating.
Raw adrenal tablets	25–50 mg daily	Helps rebuild adrenal glands exhausted after long-term substance abuse.

Homeopathic Therapy

There are several homeopathic remedies that can be helpful during the withdrawal period. To use them, put 4 pellets of 30c (or 30x) potency under your tongue and let them slowly dissolve. Repeat four times daily. Refrain from eating or drinking for ten minutes before or after using homeopathic tablets.

- *Aconitum napellus,* for restless people who toss about during withdrawal and suffer from anxiety.
- *Arsenicum album,* for those with a tendency toward vomiting or diarrhea who suffer from despair and restless agitation and don't want to be left alone.
- *Capsicum,* for those with an upset stomach, intense cravings, and delirium. It's especially helpful for recovering alcoholics.
- *Ignatia,* for those suffering from changeable symptoms that include chills, thirst, and sensitivity to pain.
- *Nux vomica,* for those suffering from twitching, trembling, and sensitivity to noise and light during withdrawal.
- *Stramonium,* for withdrawal so severe that convulsions, hallucinations, incessant talking, swearing, and lewd behavior occur.
- *Zincum metallicum,* for twitching, depression, irritability, and restlessness during withdrawal.

Flower Essences

Several Bach flower essences are appropriate for the cleansing and rebuilding that comprise withdrawal:

- **Crab apple** helps those who feel "unclean" feel more at peace.
- **Hornbeam** promotes inner vitality.
- **Larch** encourages self-confidence.
- **Walnut** aids in the release of pain of separation from an addiction.

Put 2 drops of any or all of the above flower essences in a glass of water and drink three or four times daily.

If you encounter crisis, anguish, pain, or fear during withdrawal, Rescue Remedy can be of tremendous help. Put 2 drops under your tongue, or mix them with a glass of water and drink.

Aromatherapy

Various essential oils can quell addictive cravings and help cleanse and rebuild the mind and body.

- **Basil** helps dispel addictive cravings.
- **Bergamot** helps relieve anxiety, depression, and compulsive behavior.
- **Clary sage** relieves panic, paranoia, and mental fatigue and helps dispel addictive cravings.
- **Geranium** relieves anxiety, depression, and stress.
- **Helichrysum** lifts depression, stress, and lethargy. It's an excellent tool for withdrawal.
- **Juniper** helps those who feel emotionally drained, anxious, and exhausted. It can also dispel alcohol cravings.
- **Nutmeg** helps dispel addictive cravings.

10

Addiction-Free for Life

Making It through Tough Times

Addictions often result from emotional distress. In trying times—characterized by stress, depression, loneliness, boredom, grief, pain, sleeplessness, fear, or anxiety—chemical substances offer a type of relief. They help a person cope with—or, as is more often the case, avoid—the emotional distress endemic to difficult periods in life.

Unfortunately, having beaten an addiction is not the same as having no addiction. You can't go back. Your body remembers and, given the chance, will retake the addiction in all its original intensity. If you're struggling to give up an addiction, or if you've already left one behind, you must find new tools for facing times of trial and emotional distress. You must learn how to cope with life stressors without chemical assistance. This chapter offers a few ideas.

Anxiety

The word *anxiety* derives from the Latin *angustia,* meaning "narrowness," "restriction," or "difficulty." Anxiety is a feeling of uneasy anticipation brought on by fear of the known or unknown. Anxiety is a natural by-product of the high-speed changeable world we live in. It's also a common side effect of withdrawal from drugs, including caffeine and sugar.

Anxiety causes shortness of breath, heart palpitations, chest tightness, trembling, sweating, dizziness, numbness, shaking, and muscular tension. Panic attacks, or cases of acute anxiety, can cause severe manifestations of these symptoms, to the point at which you may feel as if you're dying. Although panic attacks rarely last longer than ten minutes, they can be very disabling.

To relieve anxiety, you must nourish the kidneys, which govern the emotion of fear, and calm the heart. Remember to breathe deeply and slowly. Feed your brain the oxygen it craves for serenity.

Nutritional Therapy

To relieve anxiety, eat foods that are calming and nourishing. Here are some examples:

- **Oatmeal and yogurt** are both high in calming calcium.
- **Lettuce** helps calm anxiety.
- **Whole grains** such as buckwheat, millet, quinoa, and brown rice all contain complex carbohydrates and are very calming.
- **Vegetables** such as sweet potatoes and winter squash are calming, warming, and naturally sweet, which can help stabilize blood sugar levels.

Avoid sugar and refined carbohydrates (see chapter 3 for more details). You want to keep your blood sugar on an even keel instead of a sugar-powered roller coaster. Interestingly, experts say that the physiological symptoms of panic attacks closely mimic those of a hypoglycemic reaction.

Minimize or completely exclude all caffeinated and alcoholic products. They can contribute to further anxiety.

Herbal Therapy

Herbal teas can be tremendously helpful in soothing anxiety. Good choices include catnip, chamomile, lemon balm, oat seed or oatstraw, and passionflower, which are all calming. In addition, try the herbs listed below:

- **Calamus root** is a natural sedative and antidepressant.
- **California poppy** is cooling, calming, nonnarcotic, and soothing to the emotional body. It calms anxiety and restlessness.
- **Hawthorn** nourishes the physical and emotional heart and the kidneys.
- **Hops tincture** can calm anxiety and aid sleep.
- **Kava kava tincture** relieves anxiety and aids sleep.
- **Oat seed or Oatstraw** helps ease acute anxiety and calms and strengthens the nerves.
- **St. John's wort** helps stabilize the nervous system, relieves anxiety, and lifts depression.
- **Siberian ginseng** relieves fatigue and depression and helps the body adapt to stress.
- **Valerian tincture** calms anxiety and stress and aids sleep.
- **Wild lettuce tincture** helps calm anxiety and restlessness and improves sleep.

Flower Essences

There are several flower essences that can help relieve anxiety.

- **Aspen** flower essence is for the person who is fearful and anxious yet doesn't know why.
- **Mimulus** flower essence is for anxiety about things not working out, as with money concerns.
- **Agrimony** flower essence helps relieve restlessness and inner anxiety.

- **Rescue Remedy** is good for all sorts of anxieties. Keep it in several convenient locations, such as your briefcase, desk, purse, and the glove compartment of your car. Use it whenever anxiety starts to come on. Two drops under the tongue is all you need.

Supplement Therapy

During difficult times in your life, you may need a "supplemental" boost to help you manage without developing undue anxiety, which can lead to addiction relapse. Here are some suggestions:

SUPPLEMENT	DOSAGE	COMMENTS
B-complex vitamins	100 mg daily	A B-complex deficiency can contribute to anxiety.
Calcium	1,000 mg daily	A calcium deficiency can contribute to anxiety.
Magnesium	500 mg daily	A magnesium deficiency can also contribute to anxiety.
Lecithin granules	1 tbsp. daily	A good source of inositol and choline, both helpful in treating anxiety. Inositol is a B vitamin that can help relieve panic disorders. Choline has a tranquilizing effect.
GABA (gamma-aminobutyric acid)	750 mg daily	Helps protect the brain from excitatory messages. Research shows it can be as helpful as the drugs Librium or Valium.

Aromatherapy

Make a sachet with an aroma that's familiar to you from your childhood. Inhale the aroma deeply whenever you begin to feel anxious.

Inhale the fragrance of essential oils that are known to relax, calm, and relieve anxiety, including basil, bergamot, chamomile, geranium, jasmine, juniper, lavender, marjoram, melissa, neroli, rose, rosemary, sandalwood, and ylang-ylang.

Other Therapies for Anxiety

Surround yourself with the color blue, which is tranquil and soothing to the spirit. Practice prayer, visualizations, and peaceful mantras to calm the spirit. Soak in a warm bath scented with calming, relaxing essential oils, herbs, or flower essences.

Get or give yourself a massage to help release tensions. Hold the thumb of one hand with the other as a calming technique. Rub the third-eye chakra center—the center of the forehead between the brows—to calm the shen, or spirit. Hold your toes, especially the middle toe, to help bring the energy down from your head and ground it.

Exercise often—in the open air whenever possible—to bring more oxygen into your body and to release the emotional and physical tension of anxiety.

Insomnia

Sleep and rest are necessary for health, healing, and sanity. But as you read in chapter 8, prescription sedatives are not the answer to insomnia. They have dangerous side effects and are often habit forming. They leave you feeling less than rested and impair clarity of thought.

The best way to deal with insomnia is to determine and change the cause.

- **Are you taking any prescription drugs?** Many drugs inhibit sleep. Antibiotics, steroids, decongestants, cold remedies, appetite suppressants, contraceptives, and thyroid medications all can make sleep difficult. If your prescription medication is making it difficult for you to sleep, ask your doctor about any alternative medications. If none is available, try some of the sleep-inducing remedies suggested below.
- **Are you getting enough exercise?** It's important to get some exercise if you want restful, deep sleep. Studies show that people who are more active in the daytime are less likely to have problems with sleep. However, don't exercise right before going to bed— that can be stimulating. Tai chi, yoga, meditation, breathing exercises, biofeedback, and guided visualizations are also effective

techniques to aid sleep. Yoga postures that are especially relaxing for the mind and body and encourage deep sleep include the Corpse, Cobra Pose, Shoulder Stand, and Mountain.

Eastern Perspectives on Insomnia

In traditional Chinese medicine sleep is the supreme tonic. Many sleep problems are related to the liver, which houses the soul. Going to bed by 10:30 P.M. allows you to be in a state of deep sleep by Liver Time (from 1 to 3 A.M.), which is helpful for healing addictions.

- **Are you relaxing in the evening?** It's important—both for your sanity and for your prospects for deep, restful sleep—that you use your evening, and especially the hour before you go to bed, to relax. *Don't* eat or drink any caffeinated products after dinner. *Don't* watch action-packed television programs or read page-turning novels right before going to bed. *Don't* pay your bills right before going to bed. *Do* take a walk after dinner. *Do* savor a bedtime mug of relaxing herbal tea (see the recommendations listed below). *Do* spend time in the evening hours enjoying conversation with loved ones instead of watching television.

- **Are you eating the wrong late-night snacks?** It has been said that "sleep doesn't interfere with digestion, but digestion interferes with sleep." Avoid eating late at night, because many foods stimulate the adrenal glands and elevate blood pressure. However, if you insist on eating late at night, the few foods that can actually aid sleep include bananas, lettuce, oatmeal, and yogurt.

- **Are you using stimulants?** For some insomniacs, any amount of caffeinated food or drink may be too stimulating, even when consumed early in the day. And don't smoke before going to bed—nicotine is a stimulant, and smokers can take longer to fall asleep than nonsmokers.

- **Are you unable to sleep because your mind is busy?** Our thoughts often keep us awake. Downloading mental baggage onto a piece of paper or engagement book before bed allows slumber to carry us to dreamland, knowing that the errands of tomorrow will not be forgotten. Journal writing before bed can help express thoughts.

- **Is your insomnia a symptom of withdrawal?** In the early stages of withdrawal from an addiction, sleeping difficulties often occur. Try to not become anxious about it. You will soon find balance again.

Getting Yourself to Sleep

When you're trying to sleep, don't allow yourself to be distracted by thoughts about work, family, or other issues. Concentrate on the in and out of your breath. While you focus on your breath, practice some sort of visualization. For example, imagine that your inhalation carries the breath down to your toes, where it gathers up physical tension. Exhalation carries the breath and that tension out of the body. Move on to the top of each foot, then each sole, then each ankle, and so on, working your way one small step at a time all the way up the legs, up the belly and chest, up the arms, up the back, and across the face.

Another breathwork technique to help you get to sleep is to get comfortable in bed and take eight breaths while lying flat on your back. Turn onto your right side and take sixteen deep breaths, then turn onto your left side and take thirty-two deep breaths. Most people are asleep before they can complete the exercise.

If you lie awake in bed for more than thirty minutes, get up. Your body must learn to associate the bed with sleeping, not lying awake. Turn on a low light—not a bright one!—and write a letter or read a book. If you choose to read, don't pick out anything action packed or otherwise enthralling.

Try removing electric clocks, stereos, electric blankets, and other electrical equipment from your bedroom. For some individuals, electromagnetic pollution can stimulate the nervous system and weaken the immune system.

Remember that light is a stimulant. If there's a lot of light shining brightly through your windows at night, consider getting heavier curtains. You can also use eye masks and earplugs to help shut out the world for a while. If you make a trip to the bathroom in the middle of the night, use a red night-light rather than turning on a bright light; the brightness will jar your senses, leaving you fully awake.

Have sex! It's relaxing, warming, and can be a pleasurable prelude to sleep.

Consider saying a prayer or giving thanks for the good things in your day. Bless those you love.

Aromatic Hydrotherapy

A warm, aromatic bath before bedtime is comforting and relaxing. Add a pound of baking soda and 7 drops of chamomile or lavender essential oil to the bathwater. Baking soda makes the water alkalinizing and sedative, while chamomile and lavender essential oils are fragrant, soothing, and relaxing. When you're done bathing, open the drain and remain in the tub for a few minutes. As the water runs out, visualize all your tensions spiraling down the drain.

Herbal Therapy

There are many herbs that can be consumed in the evening to aid sleep. Focus on herbs that function as nervines (nourishing the nervous system) and as sedatives (calming the central nervous system during times of stress). Here are some good choices:

- **Chamomile** is a natural sedative that also calms anxieties and deters nightmares.
- **Hops** are a reliable natural sedative that also calms restlessness.
- **Kava kava** encourages sound sleep and calms fears and anxieties.
- **Passionflower** is a natural sedative and promotes sound sleep.
- **Skullcap** is a sedative and a nerve tonic.
- **Valerian** is another natural sedative that also functions as a muscle relaxant.

You can also make a dream pillow, which is simply a sachet about five by five inches square filled with hops. Just slip it inside your pillowcase, and the calming aroma will help you slumber soundly.

Supplement Therapy

Deficiencies in the B-complex vitamins can be a factor in poor sleep. If you're suffering from insomnia, try taking a regular daily B-complex supplement.

Calcium-magnesium supplements help nourish the nerves. Take one just before going to bed to promote sound, restful sleep.

Depression

It would be pointless to treat addiction without addressing depression. In many—if not most—cases, depression is a contributing factor to addiction. And vice versa—sometimes substance abuse is a causative factor in depression.

Many of us have experienced bouts of depression as a reaction to a difficult life circumstance or a traumatic event. Others suffer from biochemical depression, or depression caused by imbalanced hormones. Whatever the case, depression can be a difficult mental state for someone struggling to give up an addiction or for a recovered addict. The extreme emotional distress opens the door to relapse.

One of the most difficult steps in overcoming depression is simply raising enough energy to do something about it. A person who is seriously depressed may lack the motivation to follow a program and may need the help and support of a friend, family member, or health professional.

If depression is severe, you may need to seek the counsel of a professional. He or she may prescribe medication for a short period of time. If you are struggling to give up an addiction or have already left one behind, you may be hesitant to take a potentially addictive prescription drug. But follow your counselor's advice. During the period while you're taking the medication, learn how to eat better, improve your living environment,

Eastern Perspectives on Depression

In traditional Chinese medicine depression results from the liver being in a stagnant condition. Depression is caused by anger, which is the result of liver energy rising and being turned inward, against the self. So paying attention to the liver should be one of the first orders of business in treating depression.

How does the liver become stagnant? In many cases repressed emotions are causative. Anger, depression, and creativity are all connected to the liver, and creativity can be a remedy for the other two conditions. Find creative outlets. Draw. Paint. Write. Sing. Scream in an empty room. Do whatever it takes to let those repressed emotions find expression.

and handle stress and anxiety. Begin an exercise program. Find a support group or a therapist whom you feel comfortable talking to. When your depression is under control and you're ready to go off medication, you'll have the tools you need to cope with—and conquer—depression.

> Serious depression can lead to thoughts of suicide. In these cases, temporary hospitalization and/or medication may be necessary. Once the severe depression has lifted, nutritional and other holistic therapies can begin.

Nutritional Therapy

Nutrition can be a valuable tool in protecting and nurturing the liver, which will relieve depression. On a physical level we literally gum up our livers by eating foods that melt at a temperature higher than that of the body, such as margarine and shortening. Even though we may not consciously choose these foods, they're often hidden in bread, cookies, crackers, chips, and fried foods. Avoid anything whose ingredients list mentions "hydrogenated oils" or "partially hydrogenated oils." It's also wise to eat sparingly of fatty foods, which make the liver work overtime.

In addition, it's important to keep blood sugar levels steady. Consume small, frequent, meals filled with complex carbohydrates. Whole grains such as buckwheat, brown rice, millet, and oatmeal are good sources. Also eat foods that improve the liver's function, such as legumes, tempeh, miso soup, onions, scallions, ginger, basil, and oregano. Other foods to focus on are those that nourish the mind and the body, including apples, artichokes, barley, burdock root, and carrots. Include some mineral-rich sea vegetables such as kelp, dulse, or wakame to nourish the thyroid and boost a sluggish metabolism. Green leafy vegetables are high in chlorophyll and help transport oxygen into the body.

Fish and chicken can be beneficial for depression, because they're rich in the amino acids that are precursors to mood-elevating neurotransmitters. Eating two ripe bananas a day is said to help the production of serotonin and norepinephrine, both natural antidepressants.

Sourness stimulates the flow of bile and helps the liver do its job better. Try drinking your water with the juice of half a lemon added to it, and eat sour-sweet berries, such as raspberries and strawberries, to bring more of the sour flavor into your diet.

♪ Antidepressant Vegetable Juice ♭

*This juice combination is highly nutritive and can compensate for
the nutritional deficiencies that contribute to depression.*

½ cup carrot juice
¼ cup celery juice
¼ cup spinach juice
2 tablespoons watercress
1 cup springwater

Combine all ingredients and drink. Repeat daily until your depression lifts.

Herbal Therapy

Herbs offer a safe and healthful alternative to antidepressant medication. Consider the following herbs to improve depression:

- **Dandelion root** improves liver function and thus can relieve depression.
- **Ginger** improves circulation and enhances lung capacity, bringing more oxygen into the body.
- **Ginkgo** improves cerebral blood flow, which can help relieve depression.
- **Hawthorn** improves the body's ability to utilize oxygen and comforts the physical and emotional heart.
- **Kava kava** encourages emotional openness and helps alleviate fear, pain, anxiety, and depression.
- **Lavender** gently lifts the spirits.
- **Lemon balm** has been used for centuries to "maketh a sad heart merrie."
- **Licorice root** helps promote feelings of peace, calmness, and harmony.
- **Motherwort** helps reduce the pangs of grief and relieves depression and exhaustion.
- **Nettle** provides a wealth of nutrients for all body systems.
- **Oat seed or Oatstraw** is a natural antidepressant that strengthens the nervous system.
- **Rosemary** is a cerebral stimulant, nervine, rejuvenative, and antidepressant.

- **St. John's wort** is one of the world's best-researched natural antidepressants. It inhibits the breakdown of several neurotransmitters, including serotonin, which helps maintain emotional stability.
- **Siberian ginseng** helps relieve debility and exhaustion.
- **Slippery elm** is highly nutritious and is helpful for convalescence. It also helps you feel calm and stable.

> Hsiao Yao Wan is a Chinese patent medicine also known as Bupleurum Sedative. It helps to improve liver stagnation, irritability, and depression. It can be purchased at many health foods stores and from most acupuncturists.

Aromatherapy

Our nasal cavities are in such close proximity to the brain that smelling essential oils can have a very quick beneficial effect on the physical and mental body. Essential oils that can help lift your spirits from depression include:

Basil	Neroli
Bergamot	Patchouli
Cinnamon	Peppermint
Clary sage	Rose
Clove	Rosemary
Geranium	Sandalwood
Lavender	Ylang-ylang
Jasmine	

Supplement Therapy

Those undergoing stress and depression may find relief from these supplements:

SUPPLEMENT	DOSAGE	COMMENTS
B-complex vitamins	50–100 mg daily	Those suffering from depression are often deficient in B vitamins, and supplementing can result in dramatic mood improvement.
Calcium	1,000 mg daily	Can relieve depression.
Magnesium	500 mg daily	Can relieve depression.
DLPA	375–750 mg daily	Stimulates endorphin and epinephrine production and inhibits breakdown of the body's natural endorphins. Particularly beneficial for depression characterized by low energy, a sense of helplessness, and low self-worth as well as depression resulting from an external factor, such as loss of a loved one. Begin with lowest possible dosage and increase gradually and only as necessary.
Tyrosine	500 mg once in the morning and once in midafternoon	A precursor for serotonin, which lifts depression and promotes a feeling of calmness. It's especially helpful for those struggling to give up an addiction to amphetamines.
SAMe (S-adenosyl-methionine)	400 mg four times daily	Elevates levels of serotonin and dopamine, resulting in improvement from depression.

Behavior Therapy

When you're trying to recover from depression, it's important to look at your spiritual, physical, emotional, mental, and environmental state. It will take a combination of all these factors to truly lift your spirits.

We know that light affects plant and animal behavior. More research is making it clear that humans are also affected by light. Light enters the retina and travels directly to the brain, specifically parts of the hypothalamus and pineal gland. The hypothalamus regulates the sympathetic and parasympathetic nervous systems, which help maintain emotional balance and govern important life functions such as sleeping and breathing. The pineal gland activates hormones based upon the light that it receives. Without light, the hypothalamus and pineal gland don't function optimally.

Modern-day humans are light deficient. Often we go to work in darkness and return home in darkness. We live by fluorescent lighting, which doesn't give us the full spectrum of sunlight. We hide our eyes behind glasses, sunglasses, and contact lenses. So make an effort so spend some time outdoors, in natural light, every day, without glasses, sunglasses, or contact lenses. If you work under fluorescent fixtures, replace the bulbs with full-spectrum lights. It's amazing what a little natural light can do for your mood.

> **Cautions**
>
> Those with phenylketonuria or those taking MAO-inhibiting drugs should avoid DLPA. Those with high blood pressure, severe liver disease, or kidney and thyroid disorders should consult with a nutritionally trained physician before taking any isolated amino acids, including DLPA. Pregnant and nursing mothers should also avoid DLPA.
>
> SAMe is not recommended for those with bipolar conditions, because it could intensify manic behavior.

Coming home to a dirty or dingy living space will dampen anyone's spirits. Do what you can to brighten where you live so that it pleases you. Delight your senses as best you can with color, beauty, aroma, flowers, and music.

Make a list of ten activities to accomplish every day (even if they're as simple as getting dressed and making the bed). Check them off one by one as you accomplish them.

Get out and exercise! Exercise wakes up the body and stimulates endorphin production. Though exercise may not cure depression, a lack of it can be a contributing factor in being depressed.

Overcoming Fatigue and Increasing Energy

Chronic fatigue can be caused by many factors, including nutritional deficiencies, poor elimination, lack of oxygen, stress, insomnia, and poor circulation. Fatigue encompasses much more than simply a lack of energy; it reflects an inner state of nervous and emotional exhaustion. To climb out of these doldrums, you must rest and nurture all your body systems.

The Power of Oxygen

If your breathing is shallow and your posture poor, you may be missing out on some of the brain-charging properties of oxygen, one of the last free remedies! Deep-breathing exercises can increase oxygen intake and enliven the body; see chapter 2 for details. Exercise is another way of increasing oxygen intake, as is spending time outdoors. So straighten up and breathe deep the breath of life!

Nutritional Therapy

Many people overeat in a quest for more energy, but this can actually make the body have to work harder. Foods high in fat definitely slow you down. Sweets, fruit juices, and caffeine offer a quick high, but they soon leave you more tired than before. Sugar and caffeine also deplete the body of needed nutrients such as the B vitamins and calcium.

For sustained energy, eat protein-rich foods such as fish and lean poultry, legumes, nuts, and seeds as well as whole grains and fresh vegetables and fruit. Some natural supplements, such as blue-green algae, spirulina, chlorella, barley grass, and wheat grass, are loaded with nutrients such as beta-carotene, iron, protein, and chlorophyll— the wonderful oxygen-transporting lifeblood of plants.

Herbal Therapy

A number of herbs help increase energy and battle fatigue.

- **Ashwagandha** is a tonic and rejuvenative herb that's also highly nutritive. It improves memory and relieves exhaustion.
- **Codonopsis** is a chi tonic and a nutritive herb. It increases the red blood cell count and helps weak people feel stronger.
- **Ginkgo** helps relax blood vessels so more nutrients can be delivered throughout the body. It also helps the brain better utilize oxygen, thereby improving alertness.
- **Ginseng** is a chi tonic; it supports exhausted adrenal glands and helps the body better utilize oxygen.
- **Hawthorn** also improves the body's utilization of oxygen.
- **Licorice** is a chi tonic and nourishes exhausted adrenal glands.
- **Nettle** is rich in nutrients, builds healthy blood, and strengthens the kidneys and adrenals.
- **Oat seed or Oatstraw** is highly nutritive and can relieve nervous exhaustion.
- **Schizandra** improves the body's utilization of oxygen, increases endurance, and improves concentration.
- **Siberian ginseng** improves mental alertness, boosts circulation, and is a chi tonic.
- **Yerba maté** brightens the mood and stimulates the nerves. It's nutritive and antioxidant.

Aromatherapy

Inhalations of geranium, lemon, and peppermint essential oils can be very effective in relieving exhaustion. Geranium is a mild adrenal stimulant, lemon encourages a sense of freshness and well-being, and peppermint is energizing and uplifting.

Stress

For a recovered addict, stress can be a precursor to relapse. And as we're all well aware, life is full of stress, whether it be a temperature change, strong emotion, or physical trauma. Even such lofty activities as skiing down a mountain, aiming for higher goals, or falling in love can take a toll on our nerves. Though stress may be unavoidable—and indeed, life without any stress would be boring!—we can come through most ordeals if our lifestyles are balanced by faith, rest, good nutrition, and exercise.

Nutritional Therapy

During tense times, you owe it to yourself to choose nutritious foods. Whole grains are rich in complex carbohydrates, help keep blood sugar levels even, and provide important B vitamins. Oatmeal and yogurt are easy to digest and rich in calming calcium. Onions contain tension-relieving prostaglandins. Other good stress-busting foods include almonds, legumes, raisins, and sunflower seeds.

Foods that will increase the negative effects of stress include alcohol, caffeinated beverages, fruit juices, and sugar.

Herbal Therapy

Taking the time to savor a cup of soothing herbal tea is a wonderful way to nourish your nerves.

- **Ashwagandha** is an adaptogen that helps support the body's response to stress.
- **Blue vervain** is a nerve-nourishing sedative.
- **California poppy** is a skeletal relaxant and effective sedative that calms restlessness.
- **Catnip** calms the nerves and relieves stress.
- **Chamomile** helps restore an exhausted nervous system and calms restlessness.
- **Ginseng** is an adaptogen; it helps the adrenal glands conserve vitamin C during times of stress and stabilizes blood sugar levels.
- **Hawthorn** can help normalize blood pressure, which can help you feel calm, and improves the body's utilization of calcium.
- **Hops** calm those with a quarrelsome nature; they relieve restlessness and are muscle relaxants.
- **Kava kava** is both a skeletal and muscle relaxant that causes you to feel pleasantly relaxed.

- **Lemon balm** is mildly hypotensive and can calm a heart that races due to nerves. It also protects the cerebrum from excessive external stimuli.
- **Licorice** induces feelings of peace and calmness and stabilizes blood sugar levels.
- **Linden** relaxes the nerves and calms spasms.
- **Oat seed or Oatstraw** is high in calcium and B vitamins and so nourishes the nervous system.
- **Passionflower** has a quieting effect upon the central nervous system, calming restlessness and stress.
- **Poria** calms hyperactivity; it's both a sedative and a tonic.
- **Siberian ginseng** helps you acclimate to the stresses of life, and it minimizes the harmful effects of stress on the body.
- **Skullcap** calms the emotions, quiets overexcitability, and stimulates endorphin production.
- **Slippery elm** helps nourish the nerves of those who feel edgy.
- **St. John's wort** calms irritability and helps heal a damaged nervous system.
- **Valerian** is a muscle and skeletal relaxant; it calms stress and reduces pain.
- **Wild lettuce** calms restlessness and hyperactivity.
- **Wood betony** was used in medieval England to treat "monstrous nocturnal visions, devils, despair, and lunacy." Nowadays it's still used to relieve stress, nightmares, and anxiety.

Supplement Therapy

During stressful periods, consider supplementing with B-complex and C vitamins. They can not only nourish the nervous system but also give you the energy you need to deal with life's problems. Also consider adding calcium, magnesium, and potassium, which help ease tension and irritability. Our requirements for these nutrients are increased during difficult times.

101 Ways to Stay Positive and Addiction-Free

1. Encourage spirituality in your life.
2. Treat all living things as spiritual beings.
3. Live life as a prayer.
4. Pray for strength, guidance, and wisdom.
5. Meditate.
6. Breathe deeply and slowly. Oxygen nourishes the brain.
7. Chant. Allow your entire being to radiate healing sounds. *Om* works well. Or use your favorite mantra.
8. Read. Read all those books you've always wanted to, but never had the time for.
9. Make your living space beautiful and joyous. Surround yourself with the healing energy of plants, colors, and aromas.
10. Keep your living space clean.
11. Look and dress in a manner that you deem pleasing and professional. This will boost your confidence in all of life's situations.
12. Unclutter your mind. Get an engagement book and write down numbers, errands, and appointments.
13. Play music that's calming and contemplative.
14. Don't listen to music that you associate with your addiction.
15. Learn to play a musical instrument.
16. Dance.
17. Face your fears.
18. Address the issue. Don't suppress the issue.
19. Make a list of all of your good characteristics. Keep it posted on your bathroom mirror. Update as often as possible.
20. Write down all your problems and brainstorm possible ways to solve them.
21. Practice visualization. Visit these tranquil places in your mind. If you're having trouble doing it on your own, invest in some of the many audiotapes available that guide listeners through visualizations.
22. Talk to a sympathetic listener.
23. If you need outside help, get it. Find a therapist with whom

you're comfortable talking. Or join a support group—they're free, widely available, and have worked for millions of people. Support groups offer the opportunity to share what matters to you with those who understand. Bring your loved ones if they're willing.

24. Heal your inner child. We sometimes need to accept that our parents did the best they could, and they themselves may have lived with great difficulty. Be willing to forgive.

25. Nurture your inner child. Read fairy tales. Blow bubbles. Laugh. Play in streams. Be silly.

26. Spend time basking in the beauty of nature.

27. Eat right.

28. Exercise! Exercise improves respiration and circulation, sends nutrients to the cells, and stimulates endorphin production.

29. Substitute good habits for bad habits. For example, if you used to smoke after dinner, go for a walk instead.

30. Slow down. Whether you're eating, talking, walking, or driving, do it slower.

31. Take up yoga or tai chi. Both relax and strengthen the mind and body.

32. Get a massage.

33. Massage your own hands, face, and feet daily.

34. Reach out to someone. Hug your child, love your mate, put your arm around a friend, or even stroke your pet.

35. Plant a garden. Gardening is a great way to affirm faith in the future and to observe the wonders of growth and life.

36. H.A.L.T.: avoid being Hungry, Angry, Lonely, or Tired. These are the conditions that can make you most vulnerable to relapse into addiction.

37. Remember that when you feel the least like going to meetings can be the time when you need most to attend them. The support of a group has more power to keep you from relapsing than you have by yourself.

38. Make a list of the places to avoid, the people to avoid, and what needs changing in your life. On the backside write down what you need to do to achieve these things.

39. Get rid of clutter in your house.
40. Drink more water to help flush toxins out of your system.
41. In all areas of your life, delegate. You don't have to do everything yourself.
42. Wear cool, pale greens and blues to help you stay calm during stressful periods. Avoid yellow, which can contribute to anxiety, and plaids and prints, which can be too busy and cause confusion.
43. Wear comfortable clothing that allows your skin to breathe and allows freedom of movement.
44. Try a relaxing bath. Light a candle, then add a few drops of essential oils such as chamomile, lavender, rosemary, and sandalwood to the bathwater. Soak and enjoy. When you're done bathing, let the water run down the drain as you visualize all your stress going with it.
45. Maintain a sense of wonderment. Every day try to go out and look at a sunrise, sunset, the moon, or the stars.
46. Read books that connect you to your highest truth of God. Read books that are uplifting.
47. Ask yourself what the best ways are to heal yourself.
48. Learn to say no.
49. Use aromatherapy in times of stress. Essential oils that relieve stress include anise, basil, bay leaf, bergamot, cardamom, chamomile, clary sage, fennel, frankincense, geranium, helichrysum, juniper, lavender, lemon, marjoram, neroli, nutmeg, orange, peppermint, rose, sage, sandalwood, spearmint, and ylang-ylang.
50. Visit an aquarium.
51. Prepare your clothes, paperwork, and perhaps lunch the night before, rather than starting your morning in a frenzy.
52. Take naps.
53. Get up fifteen minutes earlier than you think you should.
54. Take care of unpleasant or difficult tasks early in the day, so the rest of your time can be spent more easily.
55. Treat yourself as you would a friend whom you love and care for. Find small ways to treat yourself—a new CD, a scarf, a

bouquet of flowers.

56. Get a set of Chinese hand balls, available at many natural foods stores. Learn to use them.

57. Each day find some positive way to reward yourself—an aromatherapy bath, leisure reading, or taking a walk.

58. If you're blessed with a beloved, make love to your partner very slowly. Allow yourself to experience greater pleasure in intimacy.

59. Learn a new craft. Creating things of beauty is great for self-esteem.

60. Smile. Relaxing your face helps the rest of your body as well as putting at ease those around you. Practice an inner radiating smile and give thanks; allow your heart to fill with love.

61. When you're heading to the bank, grocery store, or anywhere else where there's likely to be a waiting line, bring a book or magazine. Smile at other people in line.

62. Do something nice for someone less fortunate than yourself.

63. Take things one at a time.

64. Don't assume that the success or failure of your children is the result of your influence.

65. Spend quality time with people you care about.

66. Avoid people who cannot honor your addiction-free lifestyle.

67. Have more fun.

68. Spend some time alone every day.

69. Write down your dreams.

70. Remember that saying yes to an addiction once makes it easier to say yes twice. Remind yourself of the advantages of giving up the addiction. Reflect on these often. If a lapse occurs, evaluate why it happened and what you could do differently. Don't allow a lapse to be a relapse. Get back on your bike. You can be wiser now.

71. Consult the oracles, such as the I Ching or tarot, with a sincere heart and open mind.

72. Put all the remedies that help you stay addiction-free and relaxed in an easily accessible location so you'll remember to take them.

73. Remember the saying: "A journey of a thousand miles begins with a single step." Make it a mantra for your life.

74. Visit hot springs.
75. Be in tune with the moon.
76. Have courage.
77. Open your heart. Give yourself to love.
78. Write poems.
79. Maintain a sense of humor.
80. Remember that your true self is beyond your body and career.
81. Enjoy beautiful food that tastes good and is wholesome. Which seems closer to God: a fresh-picked peach or a bag of fried pork rinds?
82. Watch movies that are uplifting.
83. Place healing crystals on your chakras.
84. Play Tibetan bowls.
85. Every day, make a chart of ten positive, healthy things you can do in a day's time. Give yourself stars for the ones you do.
86. Celebrate!
87. Be compassionate toward those still struggling with addictions.
88. Put out a birdfeeder. Purchase a pair of binoculars and a bird identification book. Watch.
89. Volunteer.
90. Send a handwritten letter to a friend every week.
91. Make homemade treats for your pet.
92. Go for long walks.
93. Make it a habit to see something new—some detail you've never noticed before—every day on your commute to work or your walk around the block.
94. Hold babies—human, feline, canine, or otherwise.
95. Bring a homemade treat—bread, cookies, a wreath—to each of your neighbors. If you don't already know, learn their names.
96. Think globally. Act locally.
97. Go on picnics with family and friends.
98. Keep your head up. Look people in the eye.
99. Be honest. Be kind.
100. Leave this earth a better place.
101. Count your blessings—every day!

11
Herbal Basics

Herbs figure prominently in beating all types of addictions. This chapter will tell you all you need to know to purchase, gather, and use them responsibly and effectively. Those new to herbs use should visit an herb shop or a natural foods store that offers supplements and ask for assistance. Herbs are available as capsules, tablets, and tinctures as well as loose and dried. Be sure to consult your physician or a professional herbalist if you have any medical conditions or take any prescription drugs. Herbs are medicines and need to be used with care!

Purchasing Herbs

If you choose to buy commercial herbs, purchase them in bulk. Cut herbs are better than powdered, because powdering causes them to lose essential oils more quickly. Store the herbs in glass jars away from light and heat. Be sure to label each jar with the name of the herb or preparation it contains, its ingredients, how to use it (especially if it's for external use only), and the date.

Gathering Herbs

Before you gather any plant from the wild, make sure you're collecting the proper species. Some safe plants have poisonous look-alikes; use a good guidebook. Be especially careful with mushrooms—a mistake can easily be fatal. Also, be sure that you're collecting the correct part of the plant. Blue elderberries are wonderful, for instance, but the leaves are toxic. Finally, know that plants that are safe for animals to ingest are not necessarily safe for humans.

Ask permission before you gather on private land. Avoid collecting plants within fifty feet of a busy road or in any areas that are sprayed or polluted.

Any known endangered species must be left alone. Whenever possible, use a similar-quality abundant plant in lieu of a rare one. And all plants should be collected so as to ensure the continued survival of the species. Here are some ways to do this:

- Vary the places that you collect from.
- Identify the grandfather or grandmother plant and leave it to ensure the continuing vitality of the species.
- Never take more than 10 percent of the plants you find. Leave some for the wild animals!
- Harvest selectively. For example, if you need only the leaves and flowers of a particular plant, take only a few tops, leaving the roots to continue their growing cycle. Such cutting can actually promote new growth. It can also be helpful to thin any plants that are growing closely together; this will leave the remaining plants with more room.
- Replant seeds as often as possible.
- Ask permission from the herbs before you harvest. Sing while you're collecting. Be joyful! Give thanks!

When and How to Gather

Different plant parts are best collected at different times—and in various ways. All parts benefit from being misted or watered the day before you harvest, if this is possible. Following are some other guidelines for your harvest:

- **Leaves and flowers** are best collected during the time of the full moon. Gather them in the morning, after the dew has dried and before the sun is too hot. Leaves are best taken when the plant is starting to flower, not after; once a plant has flowered, its energy moves out of the leaves and into the flowers. It's kinder to take a whole leaf than to tear it.

> Echinacea is harvested only after three years; ginseng, after seven years.

- **Seeds and fruits** are collected when ripe.
- **Roots** are said to be best collected during the time of the new moon. Perennial or biennial roots are best collected in the fall of their first year or the spring of their second year. Cover the hole left when you're done—and if you can, use the opportunity to sow a few of the plant's ripe seeds!
- **Bark** is best collected in the spring or fall. It separates more easily after a spell of damp weather. Never girdle a tree; this will impair the sap's ability to rise, and can be fatal to the tree.
- **Gums and resins** are best collected in hot, dry weather.

Drying and Storing

Fresh herbs that aren't used immediately need to be dried and stored. Begin by sorting through your botanicals; any plant parts you don't need can be used as mulch, as compost, or in herbal baths. Roots should be well scrubbed, and larger ones can be cut in half for quicker drying.

Dry all plant parts in the shade. You can spread them out on a nylon or stainless-steel screen, or in a clean shallow box. Or place them loosely in a paper bag and leave them in a warm room until they're dry. Many herbs can be hung to dry with loop strings in an attic or warm room. Allow air to circulate.

Herbs should be stored as soon as they're brittle. Being careful not to crush the herbs to a powder, place them in labeled and dated

> **Herb Grinding Tip**
> If you ever need to grind resinous or sticky herbs, first place them in a freezer for a few hours. Once they're frozen they'll shatter easily in a blender or grinder. It helps if you put the blender or grinder in the freezer, too. Still, some herbs, such as saw palmetto, are just too hard to powder at home.

glass jars, and store the jars away from heat and light. Before using any final herb preparation, check its quality: it should taste and smell like the original plant. And remember that no amount of elaborate equipment or preparation will make up for poor-quality botanicals.

Herb Dosage Guidelines

All things are poison and nothing is without poison. It is the dosage that makes a thing poisonous or not.

—*Paracelsus*

There are no hard-and-fast rules governing herb dosages. Every person and every situation should be considered individually before dosage is determined. Still, the following guidelines may be helpful in this process:

- Large people need more than small people. Women may need less than men.
- After age sixty, use one-half to one-third as much herb per dose.
- For an acute or serious illness, a dosage can be taken every one or two hours—except, of course, while you're sleeping. Rest is good medicine in its own right!
- For a chronic illness that comes and goes, three or four times daily makes an effective therapeutic dosage.
- Some herbalists like to "pulse" their remedies by giving them for ten days, then taking three days off. Continue this cycle for chronic conditions. Pulsing helps the body acclimate and learn to respond even without the herbs. Another way of pulsing is to take your remedies for six days a week and rest on the seventh. Every two or three weeks, take a three-day break.

Handy Herbal Equivalents
1 cup of tea = 1 dropperful of tincture = 2 capsules

- If you're using high doses of herbs or supplements, do so only after consulting with a competent health professional.

Homeopathic Dosages

The best way to determine dosages of homeopathic remedies is to consult with a homeopath in your area. If this isn't possible, many health foods stores carry or can special-order remedies for you. These remedies are generally taken as 4 pellets under the tongue three or four times daily. It's best to take them with a "clean mouth"—that is, don't eat or drink anything for ten minutes on either side of the dose. Potencies of 30x or 30c are the most commonly recommended. If you don't see results within a week, you likely didn't select the correct remedy; talk to a homeopath.

Flower Essence Dosages

Flower essences are usually taken as 7 drops under the tongue, three times daily. They're best used in conjunction with prayer and meditation, visualizing what you want to create.

If you purchase flower essences in the form of mother tinctures, these should be diluted before use. Place 3 drops of the mother tincture in a clean amber-glass dropper bottle, then fill it with springwater. If you're going to keep the remedy for more than two weeks, add a tablespoon of brandy as a preservative. Up to six flower essences can be combined in one bottle.

Herbal Preparations

Herbal Teas

In addition to their many medicinal benefits, teas are soothing and warming. They give us the opportunity to taste the many flavors of plants. And drinking a cup is a lovely way to take a break in our busy days to sip and savor—and know that we're nourishing our nervous systems.

Herbal tea bags are convenient, but not all herbs are available in bags. If you are new to herbs and feel a bit intimidated by loose herbs, try any of the following options:

- **Infusion (for leaves and flowers).** In a nonreactive pot bring 1 cup of springwater to a boil and remove from the heat. Add

1 heaping teaspoon of dried herb or 2 heaping teaspoons of fresh. Cover and let sit for at least 10 minutes. Strain. This is also known as a tisane.

- **Decoction (for roots and barks).** In a nonreactive pot simmer together 1 heaping teaspoon of dried herb (2 heaping teaspoons of fresh) and 1 cup of springwater, covered, for 20 minutes. Strain. If a root is particularly high in volatile oils (such as ginger or valerian), it's better to infuse rather than boil it. Some roots can be used a second time.

- **Sun tea—or moon tea!** For sun tea, place 1 heaping teaspoon of dried herb (or 2 heaping teaspoons of fresh) per 1 cup of springwater in a covered glass jar; for moon tea, use an open glass bowl. Let the mixture sit outside to collect radiant energy for about three to four hours. Drink moon tea first thing in the morning.

- **Cold infusion.** Add 4 teaspoons of dried herb (or a scant 3 tablespoons of fresh) to 2 cups of cold water and let soak overnight. Strain and heat to drinking temperature, if desired. Herbs that lend themselves well to cold infusions include: anise, hyssop, basil, catnip, scented geranium, honeysuckle flowers, jasmine flowers, lavender, lemon balm, lemon verbena, marjoram, orange blossoms, rose petals, and pineapple sage.

> **Tea-Making Tips**
> - Keep a recipe file.
> - Make small batches the first time around.
> - Avoid using aluminum and copper equipment; choose nonreactive materials such as glass, stainless steel, or unchipped enamel.
> - When your tea is done, return the herbs to the earth by adding them to your compost or garden.

Herbal Tinctures

Tinctures are easy to store and use. They're traditionally started on the new moon so that the moon's energy can draw out the herbs' properties. Making a tincture involves soaking herbs (known as the mark) in a liquid (known as the menstruum) for a month or longer. Various menstruums can be used, but the process used in each case is the same:

1. Prepare the herbs by chopping or grinding. (You can tincture several herbs together if you like.)

2. Put the herbs in a jar and add enough menstruum to cover them by about an inch.
3. Shake daily.
4. After a month, strain the tincture, first through a strainer and then through a clean, undyed cloth. Squeeze tightly or press on the herbs with a potato ricer.
5. Bottle the strained menstruum in amber-glass jars. (The mark can be composted.) Be sure to label and date each jar, and store away from heat and light.

> **Tincture-Making Tip**
> When a recipe calls for "parts," these are measured by weight, not by volume.

Take tinctures by putting 1 dropperful in a bit of hot water and drinking.

You can choose your menstruum based on the herbs you're using and the benefits you're looking for. Here are some guidelines to consider:

- **Alcohol** helps preserve the herbs while extracting both their water-soluble and their alcohol-soluble properties. Alcohol must be at least 50 proof to have good preservative qualities. Vodka is the purest grain alcohol; brandy is another good choice. Alcohol is ideal for extracting fats, resins, waxes, and most alkaloids, but it doesn't extract polysaccharides effectively. Tinctures made in alcohol will last for many years. Alcohol tinctures are not suitable for those with alcohol addictions who are wanting to quit or stay "dry."
- **Vegetable glycerin** is the best menstruum for those who are alcohol intolerant, as well as for children and pregnant or nursing mothers. Glycerin is both a solvent and a preservative; its effectiveness lies somewhere between that of water and that of alcohol. It's also naturally sweet, pleasant tasting, and helps extract mucilage, vitamins, minerals, and tannins from plant material—but not resins. When diluted, it's also slightly antiseptic, demulcent, and healing. Tinctures made from glycerin are known as glycerites, and they're usually prepared using

1 part water to 2 parts glycerin. Glycerites have a shorter shelf life than alcohol tinctures—about one to three years.

- **Apple cider vinegar,** preferably organic. Look for a vinegar with about 5.7 percent acetic acid; this will impart a long shelf life. It's also a digestive tonic and can be used to season food. Warm the vinegar before you pour it over the herbs. Avoid using a metal lid, which can rust. Vinegar tinctures have a shelf life of six months to four years.

Herbal Capsules

Herbs can be powdered in a blender and put in capsules. Health foods stores offer empty capsules—both gelatin and vegetarian—for you to fill with mixtures of your own. You can do this by hand; there are also machines available that will fill about fifty capsules at once.

Capsule Sizes

- A size 0 capsule contains 400 to 450 milligrams.
- A size 00 capsule contains 500 to 600 milligrams.
- A size 000 capsule contains 650–850 milligrams.

Herbal Aromatherapy Inhalations

To make an aromatherapy nasal inhaler, add 5 drops essential oil to $1/4$ teaspoon kosher salt. Place the ingredients in a small glass vial with a lid. Open and inhale as often as needed.

Herbal Baths

Herbal baths are not only fragrant but also therapeutic. There are several ways to prepare one.

- Tie a couple of handfuls of your herbs of choice into a washcloth and secure with a strong hair tie. (Rubber bands may melt.) Place the herb-filled cloth in the bath as you fill the tub with hot water. (You are essentially making a tea in the tub!) When full, turn off the faucet and wait for the water to cool. When the temperature is right for you, get in and enjoy. You will absorb some of the properties of the herbs through your skin.

- Prepare a large pot of tea on the stove (see Herbal Teas, above) and strain it into the tub.
- One of the simplest methods is to fill the tub and add 5 to 10 drops of one essential oil—perhaps chamomile. Adding the oil after the tub is full will minimize evaporation. Close the shower curtain while you soak to help hold in the volatile oils.

Overdose First Aid

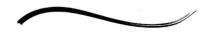

Drug and alcohol overdoses can be fatal. Slow pulse, breathing difficulty, hallucinations, pupil dilation, pale skin, sweating, vomiting, and unconsciousness are all indications of an overdose. If you suspect that someone has overdosed, you must act quickly.

Ask the victim what's going on and what he has taken as soon as possible, in case he loses consciousness. Loosen his clothing to help keep airways open; open a window to let in fresh air. Keep the patient calm. Do not allow him to take anything else. If inhalants are involved, be sure the victim is no longer exposed to any toxic vapors, and avoid lighting a match. Keep the victim away from crowds, bright lights, intense movement, and loud noises—all can worsen the crisis. He's likely to be disoriented, so watch carefully to prevent him from injuring himself.

If the patient is conscious, give her a teaspoon of charcoal or two charcoal capsules in a glass of water. If she has overdosed on alcohol, barbiturates, tranquilizers, or opiate derivatives, give strong black tea or coffee as a stimulant. Should she deteriorate or fail to improve within about five minutes, call 911.

If the victim is semiconscious, try lightly slapping him with a cold wet towel and getting him to stand. If he loses consciousness, loosen restrictive clothing and place him in the recovery position. Gently roll or move the victim on his side, with the head tilted enough to ensure that any vomitus can be expelled and the airways remain clear. Keep his mouth open and make sure his tongue is not blocking the airway. The arm touching the ground should be straight out at 90 degrees; the other arm should be bent over the chest. The leg that is not touching the ground should be bent gently at the knee. If breathing stops, use a finger to clear any obstructions from his throat or mouth; give CPR if you're properly trained. If he's having convulsions, do not administer anything or induce vomiting. Wait until the convulsions have subsided, then place the victim in the recovery position so fluids can drain from his mouth. If vomiting occurs, make sure the patient is positioned at an angle where vomit can be expelled without causing choking.

All overdose victims should receive prompt medical attention. If the patient cannot be roused, is unconscious, is diabetic, has sustained serious injuries, or may have combined drugs with alcohol, call for an ambulance. Send along a sample of any vomit, drugs, syringes, or containers; these may help medical personnel determine what has been taken. Keep the victim cool and calm until help arrives. Encourage her to breathe.

The most likely drugs to cause an overdose include heroin, morphine, tranquilizers, barbiturates, alcohol, and inhalants such as sniffed glue. Barbiturates can cause confusion; users may accidentally take another dose, forgetting that they already took some. Mixing drugs or combining drugs with alcohol is especially dangerous.

Once the crisis is past, vitamin C can help neutralize toxins in the body. An overdose should be a wake-up call to deal with your addiction now.

Resources

allGoode Organics
P.O. Box 61256
Santa Barbara, CA 93160-1256
Phone: (800) UNITEAS
E-mail:
Rob@allgoodeorganics.com
Web site:
www.allgoodeorganics.com
Offers SereniTea to calm nerves,
PuriTea to aid in detoxifying the
body, and SobrieTea to help you
get and stay substance-free.

PharmChem
3925 Bohannon Drive
Menlo Park, CA 94025
Phone: (415) 328-6200
Identifies samples of street drugs.
Send $15 money order or cash
with a random identification
code of five numbers and a covering letter. Three days after the
company receives your sample,
you can call for results.

Tools for Exploration
4460 Redwood Highway, Suite 2
San Raphael, CA 94903
Phone: (415) 499-9050 or
(800) 456-9887
Fax: (415) 499-9047
Sells Brain Machines, full-
spectrum lights, positive tapes,
and more.

Mountain Spirit Tapes
P.O. Box 4589
Boulder, CO 80306
Phone: (303) 449-8412
Makes guided visualization
tapes for quitting smoking,
weight loss, and stress relief.
Diana Keck, a member of the
American Psychotherapy
Association, also does phone
consultations and then
designs tapes tailored to your
personality. Call or write for
a catalog.

Horizon Herbs
P.O. Box 69
Williams, OR 97544-0069
Phone: (541) 856-6704
Fax: (541) 846-6233
Web site:
www.chatlink.com /~herbseed
Offers common and unusual
medicinal herb seeds.

Earth Essential
P.O. Box 35284
Sarasota, FL 34242
Phone: (800) 370-3220 for cata-
log requests and orders only;
(941) 346-3220 for customer
service
Essential oils for aromatherapy.

Zen Alarm Clock
Phone: (800) 779-6383
Web site:
www.now-zen.com
Sells clocks that wake you up
gently with harmonious bells and
positive affirmations.

HerbPharm
P.O. Box 116
Williams, OR 97544
Phone: (800) 348-4372
Makes an herbal tincture formula
called Avena/Skullcap Com-
pound for drug withdrawal.
(It's not to be used for alcohol
withdrawal, however, because it
contains alcohol.)

Bach Flower Essences
461–463 Rockaway Avenue
Valley Stream, NY 11580
Phone: (516) 593-2206

Pegasus Flower Essences
P.O. Box 228
Boulder, CO 80306
Phone: (800) 527-6104

**Rocky Mountain Center for
Botanical Studies**
P.O. Box 19254
Boulder, CO 80308-2254
Phone: (303) 442-6861
This herb school—where I and
many others teach—offers one-,
two-, and three-year programs.

**American Herbalists
Guild**
1931 Gaddis Road
Canton, GA 30115
Phone: (770) 751-6021
Fax: (770) 751-7472
Web site:
www.healthy.net/herbalists
Contact the guild to find profes-
sional herbalists in your area.

Alcohol 24-Hour Hotline
Phone: (800) ALCOHOL

**Al-Anon Family Group
Headquarters**
115 East 23rd Street
New York, NY 10010
Phone: (800) 356-9996
A resource group for the family
and friends of alcoholics.

Alcoholics Anonymous
World Service
P.O. Box 459
Grand Central Station
New York, NY 10163
Phone: (212) 870-3400

American Society of Addiction
Medicine
Phone: (301) 656-3920

American Council on
Alcoholism
Phone: (800) 527-5344
Web site:
www.aca-usa.org

American Anorexia/Bulimia
Association, Inc.
293 Central Park West, Suite 1R
New York, NY 10024
Phone: (212) 501-8351

Al-Anon/Al-Ateen
1600 Corporate Landing
Parkway
Virginia Beach, VA 42345
Phone: (804) 563-1600 or
(800) 344-2666

National Institute on Drug and
Alcohol Abuse
P.O. Box 34443
Washington, DC 20043
Phone: (301) 443-3860 or
(800) 662-HELP
Web site: www.niaaa.nih.gov

Center for Addiction and
Alternative Medicine Research
914 South Eighth Street
Minneapolis, MN 55404
Phone: (612) 347-7670
Fax: (612) 347-7669

Center for Substance Abuse
Treatment National Drug and
Alcohol Treatment Referral
Service
(800) 662-HELP

Cocaine Hotline
Phone: (800) COCAINE

Drug Free for a New Century
Hotline
Phone: (800) 487-4890
Web site: www.samhsa.gov

Food Addicts Anonymous
4623 Forest Hill Boulevard,
Suite 109-4
West Palm Beach, FL 33415
Phone: (561) 967-3871

Gamblers Anonymous
National Service Office
P.O. Box 17173
Los Angeles, CA 90017
Phone: (213) 386-8789

Health Recovery Center
3255 Hennepin Center South
Minneapolis, MN 55408
Phone: (612) 857-7800 or
(800) 9-HEROIN

Marijuana Anonymous World
Services
P.O. Box 2912
Van Nuys, CA 91404
Phone: (800) 766-6779 or
(888) MARIJUANA

National Acupuncture
Detoxification Association
NADA Clearinghouse
P.O. Box 1927
Vancouver, WA 98668-1927
Phone: (360) 260-8620

Narcotics Anomymous
World Service Office
16155 Wyandotte Street
Van Nuys, CA 91406
Phone: (818) 780-3951

National Council on
Alcoholism and Drug
Dependence Hopeline
Phone: (800) 622-2255;
(212) 206-6770; or
(in New York) (212) 979-1010

National Alliance for the
Mentally Ill
Phone: (703) 524-7600 or
(800) 950-6264

Overeaeaters Anonymous
P.O. Box 988
Hermosa Beach, CA 90254-0988
Phone: (310) 374-8533

Hazelden Educational
Facility
Box 176
Center City, MN 55012
Phone: (800) 328-3330
Books, pamphlets, and a treat-
ment center for drug and alcohol
addiction.

Rational Recovery
Phone: (916) 621-4374

Recovery Systems
Phone: (415) 383-3611

Sex Addicts Anonymous
Twin Cities S.A.A.
P.O. Box 3038
Minneapolis, MN 55403

Smokenders International
Phone: (800) 823-1126

Spender Menders
P.O. Box 15000-156
San Francisco, CA 94115
Phone: (415) 773-9754

Toughlove
Phone: (800) 333-1069

Women for Sobriety
P.O. Box 618
Quakertown, PA 18951
Phone: (800) 333-1606

Multidisciplinary Association
for Psychedelic Studies
(MAPS)
2105 Robinson Avenue
Sarasota, FL 34232
Phone: (941) 924-6277
Web site: www.maps.maps.org
Publishes an excellent journal on
psychedelic research, including
articles on addiction therapy.

Glossary

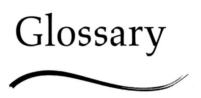

Acetaldehyde This toxic substance is the first step in the breakdown of alcohol.

Acetylcholine A neurotransmitter of the central and peripheral nervous system.

Adaptogen An agent that through hormonal response increases body's resistance to stress and aids adaptation.

Alcohol dehydrogenase A liver enzyme that helps convert alcohol into acetaldehyde.

Alterative An agent that alters your condition by increasing blood flow to tissues, detoxifying restoring body functions, aiding assimilation, stimulating metabolism, and/or promoting waste and excretion.

Analgesic An agent that relieves pain.

Anaphrodisiac An agent that curbs sex drive.

Anesthetic An agent that deadens sensation.

Anodyne A strong pain reliever that lessens nerve excitability at nerve centers.

Anticatarrhal An agent that reduces mucus.

Antiemetic An agent that counteracts nausea and vomiting

Antioxidant An agent that prevents damage from free radicals—unpaired molecules that we're exposed to through environmental pollutants.

Antispasmodic An agent that eases muscles, cramps, and psychological stress; pushes out wind; and calms energy.

Antitussive An agent that relieves coughing.

Aphrodisiac An agent that increases sexual desire and potency.

Aromatic An agent that's fragrant, pungent, and often stimulating to the digestive tract; it can improve the flavor of bitter herbs.

Bitters An agent that stimulates the flow of digestive, pituitary, liver, and duodenum secretions; clears heat; and aids digestion.

Cardiotonic An agent that benefits the heart.

Catecholamines Amines such as epinephrine and norepinephrine that have sympathomimetic activity concerned with nerve transmission, vascular tone, and other metabolic activities.

Chi Vital energy, life force. Found in all living organisms, chi is invisible, formless, tasteless, and odorless. It's extracted from food and air, then circulated throughout the body's meridians.

Cholagogue An agent that promotes bile flow from the liver and aids the breakdown of fats.

Choleretic An agent that prevents excessive bile production.

Delirium tremens Tremors, psychomotor agitation, confusion, sleep disorders—all symptoms associated with withdrawal from alcohol and some drugs.

Demulcent An agent that soothes irritated tissue of the throat as well as the gastrointestinal system. This effect is usually due to the plant's content of mucilage, a soothing, slippery substance that lubricates and heals.

Depressant An agent that lessens nervous system activity.

Diaphoretic An agent that promotes perspiration by relaxing pores and increasing elimination through the skin.

Diuretic An agent that increases the secretion and expulsion of urine and excess fluids by promoting activity of the kidneys and bladder.

Dopamine A crystalline amino acid that is a precursor to norepinephrine and other neurotransmitters.

Dosha Literally "fault" or "mistake," a Dosha is one of three forces said in Ayurvedic medicine to bind the elements into the body type of living flesh. There are three Doshas—Vata, Pitta, and Kapha.

Eicosanoids Superhormones made by every living cell in the human body; prostaglandins are eicosanoids.

Emetic An agent that induces vomiting.

Endorphins Brain neurotransmitters that help provide pleasure, pain relief, loving feelings, and psychological calm. They're the body's natural opiates.

Enkephalin A naturally occurring protein that has a morphinelike activity.

Euphoric An agent that induces a sense of buoyancy and joyfulness.

Expectorant An agent that promotes the discharge of mucus from respiratory passages.

Free radicals Unpaired molecules that we're exposed to through environmental pollutants; they can cause cellular damage.

GABA (gamma-aminobutyric acid) A brain neurotransmitter that aids in calmness and relaxation. The body's natural sedative, GABA minimizes excitatory messages to the brain.

Hallucinogen An agent that can induce hallucinations.

Hepato-tonic An agent that strengthens and tones the liver.

Hypnotic An agent that induces deep nerve relaxation and a healing sleep state.

Hypotensive An agent that lowers high blood pressure.

Kapha A Dosha corresponding to the mind-body structure. Derived from water and earth, it's considered the heaviest Dosha. Kapha makes the bones and muscles, cell walls, and basic body structure.

Laxative An agent that stimulates bowel action.

Mucilaginous Lubricating, soothing, and healing.

Mucolytic An agent that breaks up mucus.

Narcotic An agent that relieves pain and induces sleep. Narcotics sometimes produce visions and offer the potential for abuse.

Nervine An agent that calms and nourishes the nerves.

Neuron A nerve cell.

Neurotransmitters Chemicals that transmit nerve messages across the brain's synapses.

Norepinephrine A neurotransmitter that creates drive, energy, and arousal; norepinephrine is considered the body's natural stimulant.

Nutritive An agent that supplies lots of the vitamins, minerals, and nutrients that help build and tone the body.

Ojas In Ayurvedic medicine these hormonelike body substances are said to transmit energy from mind to body and contribute to immunity.

Pitta A Dosha associated with fire and heat. Pitta helps turn food into energy through digestion, and it metabolizes water and air.

Receptor site A location in the nervous system where a neurotransmitter or drug binds.

Rejuvenative An agent that renews body, mind, and spirit; it can slow the aging process, counteract stress, and increase endurance. Rejuvenatives are usually tonics.

Restorative An agent that helps rebuild a depleted condition and restores normal body functions.

Sedative An agent that slows body action and strongly quiets nerves.

Serotonin A brain neurotransmitter that creates emotional stability, confidence, and pain tolerance. Serotonin also aids restful sleep, improves self-esteem, prevents cravings for sugar and alcohol, and helps prevent nighttime depression and worry.

Stimulant An agent that quickens various body actions, improves energy and circulation, and warms the body. It's helpful for cramps and coldness.

Synapse A place where nerve impulses are transmitted from one neuron to another.

Thermogenic An agent that improves metabolism by warming the body and improving circulation.

Tonic An agent that promotes general health and well-being, improves any organ system, and builds energy, blood, and chi.

Vata A Dosha that governs circulation and the digestive process. Derived from both air and space, it can be unpredictable and always in motion—like the wind.

Vulnerary An agent that encourages wound healing by promoting cellular growth and repair. It's applied to minor external wounds.

Bibliography

Books marked with an asterisk (*) are especially helpful.

Adams, Ruth. *The Complete Home Guide to All the Vitamins.* New York: Larchmont Books, 1976.

*Balch, James F., M.D., and Phyllis Balch. *Prescription for Nutritional Healing.* Garden City Park, N.Y.: Avery Publishing, 1990.

Balick, Michael J., and Paul Alan Cox. *Plants, People and Culture: The Science of Ethnobotany.* New York: Scientific American Library, 1996.

Benowicz, Robert J. *Vitamins and You.* New York: Berkeley Books, 1983.

*Black, Dean. *Addictions: Why They Enslave Us, How to Break Free.* Springville, Utah: Tapestry Press, 1990.

Bland, Jeffrey, M.D. *Nutraerobics.* San Francisco: Harper and Row, 1985.

Bloomfield, Harold, M.D. *Healing Anxiety with Herbs.* New York: HarperCollins, 1998.

Burton Goldberg Group. *Alternative Medicine: The Definitive Guide.* Tiburon, Calif.: Future Medicine Publishing, 1997.

*Butler, Gillian, and Tony Hope, M.D. *Managing Your Mind.* New York: Oxford University Press, 1995.

Carper, Jean. *Food: Your Miracle Medicine.* New York: HarperCollins, 1993.

Cass, Hyla, M.D., and Terrence McNally. *Kava: Nature's Answer to Stress, Anxiety and Insomnia.* Rocklin, Calif.: Prima Press, 1998.

Cass, Hyla, M.D. *St. John'swort: Nature's Blues Buster.* Garden City Park, N.Y.: Avery Publishing, 1998.

Castleman, Michael. *The Healing Herbs.* Emmaus, Penn.: Rodale Press, 1991.

Chaitow, Leon. *The Body/Mind Purification Program.* New York: Simon and Schuster, 1990.

*———. *Amino Acids in Therapy.* Rochester, Vt.: Healing Arts Press, 1988.

*Chopra, Deepak, M.D. *Overcoming Addictions.* New York: Crown Publishers, 1997.

Clark, Linda. *Linda Clark's Handbook of Natural Remedies for Common Ailments.* New York: Pocket Books, 1977.

*Colbin, Annemarie. *Food and Healing.* New York: Ballantine Books, 1986.

Colgan, Michael, M.D. *The New Nutrition.* Encinitas, Calif.: C.I. Publications, 1994.

Cunningham, Donna, and Andrew Ramer. *Further Dimensions of Healing Addictions.* San Rafael, Calif.: Cassandra Press, 1988.

———. *The Spiritual Dimensions of Healing Addictions.* San Rafael, Calif.: Cassandra Press, 1988.

Cunningham, Scott. *The Magic of Food.* Saint Paul, Minn.: Llewellyn Publications, 1996.

Curtis, Susan, Romy Fraser, and Irene Kohler. *Neal's Yard Natural Remedies.* New York: Penguin, 1988.

*Davis, Patricia. *An A–Z Aromatherapy.* New York: Barnes and Noble Books, 1995.

Deann, Ward, M.D., and John Morgenthaler. *Smart Drugs and Nutrients.* Santa Cruz, Calif.: B&J Publications, 1991.

Deaton, John, M.D. *Woman's Day Book of Family Medical Questions.* New York: Random House, 1979.

De Rienzo, Paul, Dana Beal, and Members of the Project. *The Ibogaine Story.* Brooklyn: Autonomedia, 1997.

De Rios, Marlene Dobkin. *Hallucinogens.* Lindfield, Australia: Unity Press, 1990.

Donsbach, Kurt W. *Dr. Donsbach's Super Health*. Huntington Beach, Calif.: International Institute of Health Sciences, 1983.

Dufty, William. *Sugar Blues*. New York: Warner Books, 1975.

Duke, James. *The Green Pharmacy*. Emmaus, Penn.: Rodale Press, 1997.

Emery, Gary, and James Campbell, M.D. *Rapid Relief from Emotional Distress*. New York: Rawson Associates, 1986.

Erasmus, Udo. *Fats That Heal, Fats That Kill*. Burnaby, B.C., Canada: Alive Books, 1993.

Escohotado, Antonio. *A Brief History of Drugs: From the Stone Age to the Stoned Age*. Rochester, Vt.: Park Street Press, 1999.

Finnegan, John, and Daphne Gray. *Recovery from Addiction*. Berkeley: Celestial Arts, 1990.

Flaws, Bob. *Arisal of the Clear*. Boulder, Colo.: Blue Poppy Press, 1991.

Fratkin, Jake. *Chinese Herbal Patent Formulas*. Portland, Oreg.: Traditional Medicine and Preventative Health Care, 1986.

*Frawley, David. *Ayurvedic Healing*. Salt Lake City: Morson Publishing, 1992.

Fruehauf, Heiner. *The Treatment of Difficult and Recalcitrant Diseases with Chinese Herbs*. Portland, Oreg.: Institute for Traditional Medicine and Preventive Health Care, 1997.

*Gardner-Gordon, Joy. *The Healing Voice*. Freedom, Calif.: Crossing Press, 1993.

Geelhoed, Glen W., M.D., and Jean Barilla. *Natural Health Secrets*. New Canaan, Conn.: Keats Publishing, 1997.

Gittleman, Ann Louise. *Beyond Pritikin*. New York: Bantam Books, 1996.

Goldbeck, Nikki, and Steve Goldbeck. *The Goldbecks' Guide to Good Food*. New York: New American Library, 1987.

Gordon, Lesley. *A Country Herbal*. New York: Gallery Books, 1984.

Griffen, LaDean. *Health in the Space Age*. Orem, Utah: BiWorld Publishers, 1982.

Grinspoon, Lester, M.D., and James B. Bakalar. *Cocaine: A Drug and Its Social Evolution*. New York: Basic Books, 1985.

Guinness, Alma E, ed. *Reader's Digest Family Guide to Natural Medicine*. Pleasantville, N.Y.: Reader's Digest Association, 1993.

Gurudas. *Flower Essences*. Albuquerque: Brotherhood of Life, 1983.

*Haas, Elson, M., M.D. *The Detox Diet.* Berkeley: Celestial Arts, 1996.

*———. *Staying Healthy with Nutrition.* Berkeley: Celestial Arts, 1992.

*———. *Staying Healthy with the Seasons.* Milllbrae, Calif.: Celestial Arts, 1981.

Hallowell, Michael. *Herbal Healing.* Bath, England: Ashgrove Press, 1990.

Harriman, Sarah. *The Book of Ginseng.* New York: Jove Publications, 1981.

Harrison, Lewis. *Help Yourself with Natural Healing.* Englewood Cliffs, N.J.: Prentice Hall, 1988.

*Harvey, Clare G., and Amanda Cochrane. *The Encyclopedia of Flower Essence.* San Francisco: Thorson's, 1995.

Hay, Louise L. *Heal Your Body.* Santa Monica, Calif.: Hay House, 1988.

Heinerman, John. *Heinerman's Encyclopedia of Healing Herbs and Spices.* Englewod Cliffs, N.J.: Parker Publishing, 1996.

———. *The Healing Benefits of Garlic.* New Canaan, Conn.: Keats Publishing, 1994.

*———. *Heinerman's Encyclopedia of Healing Juices.* West Nyack, N.Y.: Parker Publishing, 1994.

———. *Heinerman's Encyclopedia of Fruits, Vegetables and Herbs.* West Nyack, N.Y.: Parker Publishing, 1988.

———. *The Complete Book of Spices.* New Canaan, Conn.: Keats Publishing, 1983.

———. *Science of Herbal Medicine.* Orem, Utah: Bi-World Publishing, 1979.

Heyn, Birgit. *Ayurvedic Medicine.* Northamptonshire, England: Thorsons Publishing, 1987.

Hoffmann, David. *An Herbal Guide to Stress Relief.* Rochester, Vt.: Healing Arts Press, 1991.

Hogshire, Jim. *Opium for the Masses.* Port Townsend, Wash.: Loompanics Unlimited, 1994.

Holmes, Peter. *The Energetics of Western Herbs, Volume II.* Boulder, Colo.: Artemis Press, 1989.

Hunt, Douglas, M.D. *No More Fears.* New York: Warner Books, 1988.

Igram, Dr. Cass. *Self Test Nutrition Guide.* Hiawatha, Iowa: Cedar Graphics, 1994.

Jampolsky, Lee. *Healing the Addictive Mind.* Berkeley: Celestial Arts, 1991.

Julien, Robert M., M.D. *A Primer of Drug Action.* New York: W. H. Freeman, 1995.

Justice, Blair. *Who Gets Sick: Thinking and Health.* Houston: Peak Press, 1987.

Karp, Reba Ann. *Edgar Cayce: Encyclopedia of Healing.* New York: Warner Books, 1986.

Keville, Kathi. *Herbs for Health and Healing.* Emmaus, Penn.: Rodale Press, 1996.

Keville, Kathi, and Mindy Green. *Aromatherapy.* Freedom, Calif.: Crossing Press, 1995.

Kilham, Christopher. *The Bread and Circus Whole Food Bible.* New York: Addison-Wesley Publishing, 1991.

*Kirschmann, Gayla J., and John D. Kirschman. *Nutrition Almanac.* New York: McGraw Hill, 1996.

Kohn, Marek. *Narcomania.* Boston: Farber and Farber, 1987.

Kushi, Michio. *A Natural Approach: Allergies.* New York: Japan Publications, 1985.

Larson, Joan Mathews. *Seven Weeks to Sobriety.* New York: Fawcett Columbine, 1992.

Lasater, Lane. *Recovery from Compulsive Behavior.* Deerfield Beach, Fla.: Health Communications, 1988.

Latimer, Dean, and Jeff Goldberg. *Flowers in the Blood: The Story of Opium.* New York: Franklin Watts, 1981.

Leggett, Daverick. *Helping Ourselves: A Guide to Traditional Chinese Food Energetics.* Totnes, England: Meridian Press, 1997.

Lehane, Brendan. *The Power of Plants.* New York: McGraw Hill, 1977.

Levin, Cecile Tovak. *Cooking for Regeneration.* New York: Japan Publications, 1988.

*Lewis, Walter, and Memory Elvin-Lewis. *Medical Botany.* New York: John Wiley and Sons, 1977.

*Liberman, Jacob. *Light: Medicine of the Future.* Santa Fe: Bear and Company, 1991.

Lieberman, Shari, and Nancy Bruning. *The Real Vitamin and Mineral Book.* Garden City Park, N.Y.: Avery Publishing, 1997.

Lockie, Andrew, and Nicola Gedded. *The Complete Guide to Homeopathy.* New York: Dorling Kindersley, 1995.

Long, Ruth Yale. *The Official Nutrition Education Association Home Study Course in the New Nutrition.* New Canaan, Conn.: Keats Publishing, 1989.

Lu, Henry C. *Chinese Foods for Longevity.* New York: Sterling Publishing, 1990.

———. *Chinese System of Food Cures.* New York: Sterling Publishing, 1986.

Lucas, Richard. *Secrets of the Chinese Herbalists.* West Nyack, N.Y.: Parker Publishing, 1978.

Lust, John. *The Herb Book.* New York: Bantam Books, 1983.

*McIntyre, Anne. *Flower Power.* New York: Henry Holt, 1996.

Michaud, Ellen, Alice Feinstein, and the editors of *Prevention Magazine.* *Fighting Disease: The Complete Guide to Natural Immune Power.* Emmaus, Penn.: Rodale Press, 1989.

Milkman, Harvey, and Stanley Sunderwirth. *Craving for Ecstasy.* New York: Lexington Books, 1987.

Miller, Benjamin F., M.D., and Lawrence Galton. *The Family Book of Preventative Medicine.* New York: Simon and Schuster, 1971.

Mills, Simon, and Steven J. Finando. *Alternatives in Healing.* New York: New American Library, 1989.

Mindell, Earl. *Earl Mindell's Food as Medicine.* New York: Simon and Schuster, 1994.

*———. *Earl Mindell's Vitamin Bible.* New York: Warner Books, 1979.

Morrison, Judith H. *The Book of Ayurveda.* New York: Simon and Schuster, 1995.

Mothner, Ira, and Alan Weitz. *How to Get Off Drugs.* New York: Simon and Schuster, 1984.

Murray, Michael, and Joseph Pizzorno. *Encyclopedia of Natural Medicine.* Rocklin, Calif.: Prima Press, 1991.

Murray, Michael T. *Encyclopedia of Nutritional Supplements.* Rocklin, Calif.: Prima Publishing, 1996.

———. *Natural Alternatives to Prozac.* New York: William Morrow, 1996.

———. *The Healing Power of Foods.* Rocklin, Calif.: Prima Publishing, 1993.

Naess, Inger. *Color Energy.* Vancouver, Canada: Color Energy Corporation, 1996.

*Nauman, Eileen. *Poisons that Heal.* Sedona, Ariz.: Mission Possible Commercial Printing, 1995.

Nuckols, Cardwell C. *Cocaine: From Dependency to Recovery.* Blue Ridge Summit, Penn.: Tab Books, 1989.

Ortiz, Elisabeth Lambert. *The Encyclopedia of Herbs, Spices and Flavorings.* New York: Dorling Kindersley, 1992.

Pedersen, Mark. *Nutritional Herbology.* Warsaw, Ind.: Wendell W. Whitman, 1994.

Pert, Candace. *Molecules of Emotion.* New York: Simon and Schuster, 1997.

*Phelps, Janice Keller, M.D., and Alan E. Nourse, M.D. *The Hidden Addiction.* Boston: Little, Brown, 1986.

Pilkington, J. Maya. *Alternative Healing and Your Health.* New York: Ballantine Books, 1991.

Pitchford, Paul. *Healing with Whole Foods.* Berkeley: North Atlantic Books, 1993.

Potter, Beverley, and Dan Joy. *The Healing Magic of Cannabis.* Berkeley: Ronin Publishing, 1998.

Prevention Magazine Editors. *The Doctors Book of Home Remedies.* Emmaus, Penn.: Rodale Press, 1990.

———. *Stopping Sickness: How to Protect and Restore Good Health.* Emmaus, Penn.: Rodale Press, 1987.

Prevention Magazine Staff. *The Encyclopedia of Common Diseases.* Emmaus, Penn.: Rodale Press, 1976.

*Radeliffe, Anthony, M.D., Peter Rush, Carol Forrer Sites, and Joe Cruz, M.D. *The Pharmer's Almanac.* Denver, Colorado: M.A.C. Printing and Publication, 1985.

*Reader's Digest Association. *Foods That Harm, Foods That Heal.* Pleasantville, N.Y.: Reader's Digest, 1997.

Reader's Digest Editorial Staff. *Magic and Medicine of Plants.* New York: Reader's Digest Association, 1986.

Reuben, David, M.D. *Dr. David Reuben's Mental First Aid Manual.* New York: MacMillan, 1982.

———. *Everything You Always Wanted to Know about Nutrition.* New York: Simon and Schuster, 1978.

Rodale, J. I., and Staff. *The Health Seeker.* Emmaus, Penn.: Rodale Books, 1971.

Rose, Jeanne. *The Aromatherapy Book.* San Francisco: Herbal Studies Course, 1992.

————. *Herbs and Things.* New York: Grosset and Dunlap, 1976.

Rosengarten, Frederic, Jr. *The Book of Spices.* New York: Pyramid Books, 1973.

Rushkoff, Douglas, and Patrick Wells. *How to Get High without Drugs.* New York: Dell Publishing, 1991.

*Sachs, Judith. *Nature's Prozac.* Englewood Cliffs, N.J.: Prentice Hall, 1997.

Sahley, Billie Jay, and Katherine M. Birkner. *Breaking Your Addiction Habit.* San Antonio, Texas: Pain and Stress Therapy Publication, 1990.

*Saifer, Phyllis, M.D., and Merla Zellerbach. *Detox.* New York: Ballantine Books, 1984.

*Salaman, Maureen. *Foods That Heal.* Menlo Park, Calif.: Stratford Press, 1989.

Salat, Barbara, and David Copperfield. *Well-Being.* Garden City, N.Y.: Anchor Books, 1979.

Samuels, Mike, M.D., and Hal Bennett. *The Well Body Book.* New York: Random House, 1973.

Santillo, Humbart. *Natural Healing with Herbs.* Prescott Valley, Ariz.: Hohm Press, 1984.

Schivelbusch, Wolfgang. *Tastes of Paradise: A Social History of Spices, Stimulants, and Intoxicants.* New York: Pantheon Books, 1992.

Schoenfield, Eugene, M.D. *Dear Dr. Hip Pocrates.* New York: Grove Press, 1968.

*Schwartz, George, M.D. *Food Power.* New York: McGraw Hill, 1981.

Sears, Barry. *Enter the Zone.* New York: HarperCollins, 1995.

Sheppard, Kay. *Food Addiction: The Body Knows.* Deerfield Beach, Fla.: Health Communications, 1989.

Shurtleff, William, and Akiko Aoyagi. *The Book of Kudzu.* Wayne, N.J.: Avery Publishing, 1985.

*Sibley, Uma. *The Complete Crystal Guidebook.* San Francisco: U-read Publications, 1986.

Smith, David, M.D., and George Gay, M.D. *"It's so Good, Don't Even Try It Once": Heroin in Perspective*. Englewood Cliffs, N.J.: n.p., 1972.

Smith, Lendon, M.D. *Feed Yourself Right*. New York: Dell Publishing, 1983.

Souter, Keith. *Curecraft*. Essex, England: C. W. Daniel, 1995.

*Stafford, Peter. *Psychedelics Encyclopedia*. Berkeley: Ronin Publishing, 1982.

Stanway, Andrew. *The Natural Family Doctor*. New York: Simon and Schuster, 1987.

Stanway, Penny. *Foods for Common Ailments*. New York: Simon and Schuster, 1989.

Stone, Thomas A. *Cure by Crying*. Des Moines, Iowa: Cure by Crying Incorporated, 1995.

*Strohecker, James, ed. *Natural Healing for Depression*. New York: Berkeley Publishing, 1999.

Stuart, Malcom, ed. *The Encyclopedia of Herbs and Herbalism*. New York: Crescent Books, 1989.

Svoboda, Robert E. *Ayurveda: Life, Health and Longevity*. New York: Penguin, 1993.

*———. *Prakuti: Your Ayurvedic Constitution*. Albuquerque: Geocom Limited, 1988.

Thomson, Robert. *The Grosset Encyclopedia of Natural Medicine*. New York: Grosset and Dunlap, 1980.

Trattler, Ross. *Better Health through Natural Healing*. New York: McGraw Hill, 1988.

*Trickett, Shirley. *Coming Off Tranquilizers*. New York: Thorson's Publishing Group, 1986.

Tyler, Varro E. *The Honest Herbal*. New York: Pharmaceutical Products Press, 1993.

Vayda, Dr. William. *Mood Foods*. Berkeley: Ulysses Press, 1995.

Verma, Dr. Vinod. *Ayurveda for Life*. York Beach, Maine: Samuel Weiser, 1997.

Wade, Carlson. *Health Secrets from the Orient*. Bergenfield, N.J.: New American Library, 1973.

Wallnofer, Heinrich, and Ann Von Rottauscher. *Chinese Folk Medicine*. New York: New American Library, 1972.

Warmbrand, Max,. *Encyclopedia of Natural Health.* St. Catherines, Ont., Canada: The Provoker Press, 1962.

Weil, Andrew, M.D. *Health and Healing.* Boston: Houghton Mifflin, 1985.

————. *Chocolate to Morphine.* Boston: Houghton Mifflin, 1983.

————. *The Natural Mind.* Boston: Houghton Mifflin, 1972.

Weiner, Michael, and Kathleen Goss. *The Complete Book of Homeopath.* New York: Bantam Books, 1982.

Weiner, Michael. *Weiner's Herbal.* Mill Valley, Calif.: Quantum Books, 1990.

Weiss, Rudolf Fritz, M.D. *Herbal Medicine.* Beaconsfield, England: Beaconsfied Publishers, 1985.

Werbach, Melvyn, M.D. *Nutritional Influences on Mental Illness: A Sourcebook of Clinical Research.* Tarzana, Calif.: Third Line Press, 1991.

Wilen, Joan, and Lydia Wilen. *Live and Be Well.* New York: Harper-Collins, 1992.

————. *More Chicken Soup and Other Folk Remedies.* New York: Ballantine Books, 1986.

Willard, Terry. *Textbook of Modern Herbology.* Calgary, Alb., Canada: C. W. Progressive Publishing, 1988.

Williams, Tom. *The Complete Illustrated Guide to Chinese Medicine.* Rockport, Mass.: Element Books, 1996.

Winek, Charles. *Everything You Wanted to Know About Drug Abuse . . . But Were Afraid to Ask.* New York: Marcel Dekker, 1974.

*Worwood, Valerie Ann. *The Fragrant Mind.* Novato California: New World Library, 1996.

————. *The Complete Book of Essential Oils and Aromatherapy.* San Rafael, Calif.: New World Library, 1991.

Zevin, Igor Vilevich. *A Russian Herbal.* Rochester, Vt.: Healing Arts Press, 1997.

Index